Advance Pr...

"*The Clean-Eating Kid* is the ultimate resour... ...usy parents who want to give their kids the most nutritious food possible – without having to make everything from scratch. (Who has time for that?!) From sneaky nicknames for sugar to what to look out for on labels to a rundown of brands you can trust, Jenny Carr has a knack for providing need-to-know info in an (ahem) easy-to-digest manner."

—**Emily Laurence**, Senior Food+Health Editor, Well+Good

"*The Clean-Eating Kid* helps families navigate the tricky world of food inflammation and starts your family on a path to healthy eating. Finally, a tool kit to help take the stress out of meal planning, holidays, and parties."

—**Colleen Wachob**, co-founder, MindBodyGreen

"Carr is on a mission to support the youngest generation as they experience healing through diet. *The Clean-Eating Kid* will show you how to make anti-inflammatory eating a *reality* for the whole family."

—**Mark Hyman**, MD, *New York Times* Bestselling Author

"If there is one thing that can make the biggest difference for the children and families I see in my practice, it's shifting to a cleaner way of eating. Most kids eat diets high in processed foods that lead not only to unhealthy weight gain, but contribute to learning, mood, and behavior challenges. Jenny Carr has uncovered the simple secret to helping kids feel and function better – remove all those sneaky inflammatory sugars! *The Clean-Eating Kid* is a practical resource that spells out exactly what to eat and why, while getting even picky eaters on board. The entire family will enjoy better physical and mental health one anti-inflammatory food swap at a time."

—**Nicole Beurkens**, PhD, Clinical Psychologist and
Board-Certified Nutrition Specialist

"Carr's conversational writing style includes personal stories and scientific facts woven together in an easily implementable format. If you are a new or soon-to-be parent, this book will be your go-to lifestyle resource. If you have picky eaters, or children with chronic health conditions, you will start reading this book and feel relief—because this book includes all the details you need, presented in a pleasant and easy to follow manner, with an emphasis on implementation. Carr provides enough scientific background for you to understand what is at issue, and then emphasizes the actions to take in your own kitchen so that you raise vibrant, healthy children and can focus the rest of your energy on living life.

It's also nice that food swaps, which improve your children's health, are easy to do and will positively impact the whole family!"

—**Alexandra Stockwell**, MD

The Clean-Eating Kid

The Clean Eating Kid

Grocery Store Food Swaps for an Anti-Inflammatory Diet

JENNY CARR

NEW YORK

LONDON • NASHVILLE • MELBOURNE • VANCOUVER

The Clean-Eating Kid

Grocery Store Food Swaps for an Anti-Inflammatory Diet

Published in New York, New York, by Morgan James Publishing. Morgan James is a trademark of Morgan James, LLC. www.MorganJamesPublishing.com

All material provided in The Clean-Eating Kid and from Jenny Carr is provided for informational or educational purposes only. The instructions and advice presented are in no way intended as medical advice or as a substitute for medical counseling. Neither this diet nor any other diet should be followed without first consulting a health care professional. If you have any medical condition requiring attention, consult with your health care professional regularly regarding the best way to adopt the anti-inflammatory diet outlined in this book. The author's references to various products are for informative purposes only and are not intended as an endorsement for those products by the author, her book, or the publisher. Statements made about products and descriptions of those products are accurate as of the writing of this book in July 2019.

Neither the author nor the publisher assumes any responsibility for errors, omissions, or contrary interpretations of the subject matter herein. Any perceived slight of any individual or organization is purely unintentional.

Brand and product names are trademarks or registered trademarks of their respective owners.
ISBN 9781642794489 paperback
ISBN 9781642794496 eBook
Library of Congress Control Number: 2019931141

Cover Design: Jennifer Stimson
Interior Design: Chris Treccani
Cover Photo of Tosh Carr: Arron Kraft
Editing: Bethany Davis and Maggie McReynolds
Author Photo: Aaron Kraft
Interior Photos: Jamye Chrisman

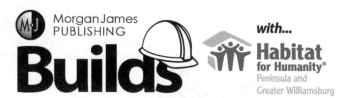

Morgan James is a proud partner of Habitat for Humanity Peninsula and Greater Williamsburg. Partners in building since 2006.

Get involved today! Visit
MorganJamesPublishing.com/giving-back

Tosh and Chloe, you are my teachers.

I am so grateful I get to be your mom.

Table of Contents

———

Foreword

Suppose you ask your friendly neighborhood pediatrician: "Doctor, what is the most important gift I can give my kids to increase their chances of living a healthier, happier, and longer life?"

Smart Doc replies, "Raise a clean-living kid!"

That's what Jenny helps you do in her book. Early on in our parenting, Martha and I realized this was the best long-term investment we could give our children. Our daughter, Hayden, announced in her wedding toast: "Thanks, Mom and Dad, for giving us kids the gift of health!"

In this invaluable guide to her practical and tasty anti-inflammatory protocol, Jenny gives readers tips and tools for preventing and alleviating the number one root cause of nearly all disease: inflammation. Her main mantra for raising a clean-eating kid is: "To avoid junk behavior and junk learning, avoid junk carbs."

Each day in my office, while counseling families suffering from inflammatory diseases, I give them one take-home tip: "Avoid sugar spikes!" In her clean-eating protocol, Jenny helps families clean their kitchens of inflammation-producing carbs and replace "chemical food" with real food. And, to help consumers outsmart food packagers, she lists all the aliases for added sugars that may appear deceiving on food labels.

A "wow!" read is how Jenny takes on Big Chem by exposing what I call "sprayed in America!" A riveting read is her exposé on how the pesticide Roundup™ – top on my neurotoxin naughty list – is polluting our food and our health. This food pollution is doubly important for children for three reasons: 1) their brains are growing the fastest at the stages in their lives when they eat the most polluted food; 2) the rapidly growing cells of rapidly growing children are particularly sensitive to chemical-food pollution; and, finally, 3) the extra fat on naturally frumpy infants and preteens are storage tanks for the chemical toxins that infect our food. If a friend inquires, "Why are you reading *The Clean-Eating Kid*?" respond, "I'm detoxing my home!"

A pleasing feature readers will enjoy is that Jenny doesn't dwell on the problems in our polluted food supply, but rather focuses on the solutions by offering shopping carts full of information about clean shopping for clean eating.

As an added perk to what you read, besides clean eating, it's so important to teach children tools to enjoy calm and clear minds. Take a deep breath and enjoy the meditation tips the author talks you through during a nice walk in the woods with your children.

Enjoy being a clean-eating family!

~ William Sears, MD, co-author of *The Dr. Sears T5 Wellness Plan: Transform Your Mind and Body, Five Changes in Five Weeks*

Introduction

———

Parenting another human, one you love more than you thought humanly possible, is quite an adventure. It means being not only your child's caregiver but also their teacher, counselor, authority figure, friend, financial consultant, cheerleader, and nutritionist. It's a big job.

For me, that job – parenting my incredible kids, Tosh and Chloe – led to my other job as an anti-inflammatory nutrition expert. As a family, we struggled at one time with chronic physical illnesses and challenging behavioral conditions. I learned everything I know about inflammation and nutrition in order to help my family move out of what were some truly scary times, health-wise, and into vibrant living. In this book, I'll teach you what I learned – simple, real-life steps you can take to help your kids be healthy and happy.

Happiness might seem like a tall order for a nutrition book to deliver. But good health isn't just about eliminating or preventing symptoms. It's about having the ability to live life on our terms, to be able to be active, engaged, and doing the things we want to do. Our youngest generation has incredible potential and possibility before them: the potential to create such goodness on our planet and the possibility of living life as they dream it to be. It is our job, as parents, to make sure they have the fundamental supports in place to do just that. Good heath is key.

At one time, inflammation was something people associated with physical injury and treated with an ice pack. Now we know that systemic inflammation, in which the body's white blood cells produce a constant response to an onslaught of damaged cells, irritants, and pathogens, is at the root of most chronic illnesses, symptoms, and conditions. And, sadly, this inflammation can predispose us to life-threatening conditions like cancer and heart disease, among many. Systemic inflammation isn't something we can treat just by placing a bag of frozen peas on a swollen area of the body. (That said, that bag of peas can be a different part of healing to reclaim our health and prevent disease. More on that later.)

That's why, as both a mom and an inflammation expert, my primary focus is helping people recover their health and melt away chronic symptoms by eliminating inflammation – and to do so without feeling overwhelmed or deprived. I've dedicated my career and research to helping others push inflammation from their bodies so they can reverse symptoms and live the day-to-day life they dream of.

Over the past decade of helping thousands of people, I've discovered that focusing on removing the toxic overload that inflammation represents is the *fastest, most effective* method to regenerate the cells in your body and experience long-lasting healing. Yet the world of nutrition is confusing and full of contradictions. One person recommends coconut oil, and another says it's bad for you. One person says nuts are a great source of protein, while another says too many can cause inflammation. As a parent, I know how difficult it can be to get your child to eat anything other than what he/she is used to. If you're going to make the effort to create a positive change in your family's diet, you definitely want to be certain that those changes will give everyone the outcome they want – with a minimum of complaining.

If you want to reverse a *chronic* symptom, know that eliminating *chronic* inflammation is key. But it doesn't have to be hard. In this book, I outline, step by simple step, exactly what to do. I also include specific tips and guidelines that will give you and your family the best bang for your buck so that you can remove the most inflammation possible without everyone feeling overwhelmed or deprived.

My family's story about the damage inflammation can do may be more dramatic than most – but it's not, sadly, unique. Inflammation is a societal and systemic issue. My heart tugs when I see the statistics showing that our youngest generation is in declining health. In fact, this is the first time in history that our youngest generations are predicted to live shorter lives than their parents, largely due to the foods today's kids are consuming. It's critical that we turn this around, that we give our kids everything they need to enjoy clear minds, confidence, and the ability to use their bodies without restriction and without subtle or debilitating symptoms.

It's time to take a stance and give our children the quality of life they deserve – but they need our help to make that happen.

In *The Clean-Eating Kid,* I've designed a streamlined approach to anti-inflammatory eating for your family that focuses on one simple food group, processed sugar. To make the biggest impact on your child's overall health, your family will learn how to swap out processed sugar for natural sugars that do not cause inflammation. By incorporating food swaps for options that taste similar but don't inflame, we get to satisfy our taste buds while simultaneously restoring health. It's a win-win!

The secret to following an anti-inflammatory diet begins with eliminating processed sugar because, when you do this, many of the top inflammatory foods fall to the wayside. There are so many treats without inflammatory ingredients, and it's important we make these available to our children so that they can experience good health without feeling deprived. In this book, you will find grocery store swaps for cake mixes, cookies, breads, pizza, and more. Anti-inflammatory eating does not mean eating kale salad every day (no offense to kale)! Instead, you can have the foods you love by swapping out the inflammatory ingredients for similar-tasting options without the inflammatory side effects. Now that's pure magic!

Replacing inflammatory foods with non-inflammatory alternatives that your kids love is the single most effective way you can help your child initiate the reversal of chronic symptoms. By following the steps in this book, you and your family will begin to melt inflammation from your bodies. Because inflammation is at the root of chronic conditions, you all will *naturally* feel better. Feeling better translates into more confidence, stronger relationships, heightened school and work focus, and improved athletic performance, to mention a few outcomes. Your family's overall sense of well-being will improve, creating rich opportunities for a beautiful life.

But knowing what to do and then actually doing it are two different things, and it's easy to get lost in the gap between the two. Let's make sure our kids don't fall into this gap. Let's take easy steps to improve their health and raise their confidence. It's simple: you teach them how to eat by how you feed yourself every day. In doing so, you make a commitment to teaching them how to enjoy longevity and vitality throughout life.

Part 1 of *The Clean-Eating Kid* will walk you through the cost of continuing to live with a chronic health condition, how you can best support your child and improve their health, and the easiest and tastiest way to push inflammation from the body. Because this book is a guide to supporting both you and your child in gaining health and vibrancy, I have added "The Clean-Eating Kid Tips" sections as a quick reference near the end of each chapter, beginning in Chapter Three and throughout the rest of the book. My intention is to create an action-oriented and easy-to-follow reference so you can make clean eating a reality for your family.

Part 2 will walk you through each aisle of the grocery store so you can see foods swaps that my family eats, which are free of the top six inflammatory ingredients and also taste great! (And because it's important for me to give you up-to-date information about new and exciting food companies, I have created a website with additional swaps that will come during the publishing of this book, so be sure to check it out at www.cleanfoodswaps. com.) Together, you and your family can improve your health while making meal prep simple and easy!

PART 1:

Renegade Researching
for Your Family

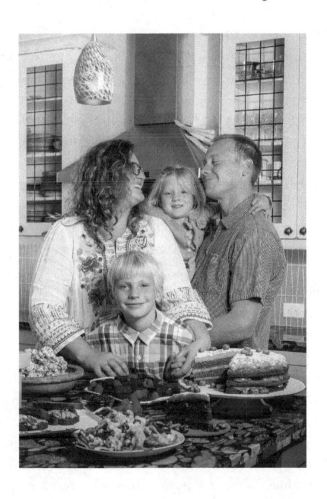

Chapter 1

The Cost

Every Mom's Dream

Isn't it amazing the way our children become our teachers? I would never have become one of the country's leading inflammation experts – something I never imagined – if not for my post-partum health challenges. Each time I figured out how to heal one of my health issues, I found that I could apply my new knowledge to helping one or both of my kids. That practice of healing, first myself and then my kids, grew to helping friends and family and then, ultimately, to helping thousands of people around the world.

This is, by the way, one of the greatest gifts that comes with clean eating. As you show up to heal yourself, you inspire so many people along the way!

I imagine that if you're reading this book, you deeply care about the health and well-being of your child. You probably also understand the connection food has to our body's ability to reverse chronic symptoms. Please know I am with you, hand in hand and heart to heart, as we take the path less traveled and create new norms of eating for our families. I am deeply touched by you joining this incredible journey with me.

I was raised in a family that valued good health. My belief, back then, was that if you ate a relatively well-balanced diet and exercised, you had your bases covered, and you could assume good health for life. That worked for a while. When I was young, exercise and a reasonably well-balanced diet were enough to keep me relatively healthy. But the food industry has dramatically changed since my childhood – and yours. What were once considered whole foods are now being turned into food-like products, commonly referred to as Frankenfoods.[1] Over the course of a few decades, systemic inflammation has dramatically risen, paralleling the rise of chronic illness symptoms in adults and children alike.

It's bad enough for us adults, but our kids are even more at risk. Theirs is the first generation to be exposed since birth to horrifying levels of toxins in our food. Their bodies are inundated with the Frankenfoods that have replaced real nutrition, leading to toxic overload and chronic inflammation. In fact, babies are now being born with an average of *a hundred* different toxins and chemicals in their umbilical cords, according to a report conducted by the environmental research and action organization Environmental Defense.[2] These toxins have been traced back to the environment as well as to consumer products and foods. Even scarier, the chemicals found are linked to serious health conditions such as cancer and brain and nervous system toxicity.

Our babies aren't even getting a fair and fighting chance to start off in life with good health and vitality. From birth, they are exposed to inflammation and toxins that come from either formula or mother's milk (if the mother is eating inflammatory foods), followed by the steady supply of the top inflammatory foods found in baby, toddler, and kid-friendly meals. The odds seem stacked against those who are most precious to us.

I understand the innate desire moms feel to give their children the best start in life. When my son Tosh was born, I knew the importance of eating organic foods, and I was determined to raise a healthy son. I gave him organic whenever I could find it, from formula and Earth's Best Organic Granola Bars to organic cereal, milk, cheese, crackers – you name it. I also exposed him to an active lifestyle and mentally made a note: "Check, Tosh will be a healthy boy. I've done my job as a mother."

I was disabused of this notion when Tosh turned six months old, and I realized he was getting more ear infections than most babies. It seemed as though he had been on antibiotics a lot, but then again, I was a new mom, and I didn't know what was normal. I chalked up the ear infections to lots of colds going around – until Tosh also started to get acid reflux. It became so severe that when Tosh ate, he would throw the food back up eight times out of ten.

Tosh was given a special diet that required I take him off organic formula and put him on a specific, acid-reflux formula made by Nestlé. I vividly remember the day the doctor told me we had to change formulas. I was devastated. I was worried that a non-organic formula would make Tosh even sicker. What I didn't realize is that both formulas, organic and non, had processed sugar, adding to the inflammation in his body.

I felt like I had already failed as a mom. Guilt flooded through every cell of my body, yet I felt my hands were tied. I didn't know what to do besides move forward with the Nestlé formula. I prayed that Tosh would still be able to remain a healthy boy.

In the months to come, Tosh's immune system became so compromised that he ended up getting every virus possible from the live vaccines given to him, including chickenpox and rotavirus, a severe virus that made everything he ate immediately come out his other end. That was particularly scary in a young baby for whom constant elimination could quickly spiral into a dire need for hydration and nutrients. Next, Tosh ended up with chronically infected tonsils and adenoids. Time and time again, Tosh was put on antibiotics, averaging a set of antibiotics nearly every other month. I cringe at this statistic now. We were wiping out the good bacteria in his gut and directly lowering his immune response to infection – and at such an early age! Yet I didn't know what else to do. I felt helpless and desperate to find a solution.

The Cost

As the doctor appointments added up, so did the prescriptions, the worry, the stress, the missed days at work, the financial shortfalls, and the emotional crashes. During Tosh's first year of life, I missed more time at work than I had during my maternity leave. Each day, I sat at home trying to do whatever I could to comfort my baby while simultaneously writing lesson plans (I was a teacher at the time) and sending emails to parents and colleagues. I was spread incredibly thin, hoping each and every day that Tosh would magically become healthy. The amount of time and energy I spent researching and trying to figure out what was "wrong" with Tosh represented a second full-time job.

Had Tosh simply gotten a few colds, as all babies do their first year of life, my experience would have been entirely different. It wasn't one specific health condition or infection that put me over the edge, but rather the *chronic, insistent, numerous symptoms* that Tosh experienced. I wanted to cry "uncle" time and time again. If only it was that easy. Instead, I did the only thing I knew at the time, which was to go from doctor to doctor and medication to medication, hoping our nightmare would soon end.

It got to the point that if Tosh caught just a common cold from daycare during this time, he would end up with a fever of 103-106 degrees (even with the use of Tylenol alternating with ibuprofen). The doctor was on speed dial and required that we call in with an hourly report to update her on Tosh's condition. If we were lucky, he would drink (but rarely eat), and the fever would pass eventually, allowing us a sigh of relief. More commonly, we would end up in the ER and spend days or weeks in the hospital, which meant Tosh receiving a lot of pricks, prods, and pokes from nurses and doctors to effectively conduct their tests.

The ear, nose, and throat specialist we consulted decided that Tosh should have his adenoids removed. They'd been chronically inflamed and infected for months and months, with antibiotics doing little to no good. His infections would heal momentarily only to give way to another infection days or weeks later. Immediately after the adenoid surgery, the doctor told us that Tosh's tonsils were the largest and most inflamed he had ever seen for any kid his age (he was then one year old). It was now the doctor's belief that many of Tosh's health issues stemmed from his chronically infected tonsils, and he recommended that we travel to Primary Children's Hospital in Salt Lake City, Utah (five hours from home) to have a pediatric specialist conduct the procedure. Can you see how one procedure can spin into needing another? This is so common in the medical world, and it leaves parents – it left us – feeling utterly helpless.

Of course, as parents who wanted the very best for our son, we jumped at the chance to "heal" Tosh once and for all. The trick: Tosh had to be healthy enough, for a long enough period of time, to schedule and conduct the surgery. So far, in Tosh's short life, he had not experienced a period of consistent good health long enough to qualify for the surgery. By the same token, we were being told that, in order to stop all of these crazy chronic health issues, we had to have his tonsils removed. It felt like we were stuck in a medieval torture chamber, knowing what could heal our son, but unable to do it because he was not healthy enough. It was rare for Tosh to go two solid weeks without infections.

My sick days were used up, my career was suffering, my adrenals were shot, my energy was on a downward spiral, and all life as I had known it, pre-kid, was over. The energy and time I once used to take care of myself were now devoted to my child, compromising my health as well as my power to care for him to the best of my ability. Not to mention, the bills were stacking up. From one hospital stay alone, we had a $28,564 bill. What a way to enter motherhood! It was certainly not the life I had imagined. I desperately combed the internet, looking for a magical cure. I didn't know yet that one actually existed – nor that I would soon learn of it in a way I couldn't have expected.

When your child has a chronic health condition, or when you have one yourself, you can fall into a pattern of living that seems, if not normal, then at least familiar. I got used to going to the doctor all the time, missing work, and paying expensive medical bills. I got used to my own self-care deteriorating, and to no longer finding the time to spend with friends. I was a former athlete, but all my athletic endeavors had ground to a halt. My career was suffering, and my energy was dwindling. I didn't realize this at the time, but having a chronically ill child was impacting every single aspect of my life.

How are your family's (or your own) health conditions impacting your life? What is the cost of not solving this health problem? It is often about far more than simply wanting to feel better. Our poor health hinders us from living life full-out.

When I asked myself the same question, I realized that for me, the cost of living with a chronic health condition went far beyond straining our financial resources – which, of course, it did. It cost me in other ways every day as well. I struggled with low energy and the inability to show up as the mom, wife, athlete, and then-teacher I wanted to be. It made me feel unworthy, and brought on an unwelcome slump into depression. I wasn't present for me, and I wasn't present for my family – and that motivated me to find another way, and I'm so grateful I did. This knowledge and lifestyle has not only helped heal my son but also helped to save my life later down the road. What a gift!

Chapter 2

The Magic Answer

Touch and Go

The longest stint we stayed in the hospital with Tosh was for one month at Primary Children's. Tosh had his tonsils removed, finally, and during recovery ended up catching RSV (Respiratory Syncytial Virus). There were two distinct times during his early years that I wasn't sure whether Tosh would make it through to see the next day. Even today, writing this, my stomach flips over, my hands get sweaty, and my heart beats fast. It was a horrible time for our family, and one that could have potentially been avoided had I known how to remove inflammation from his life.

Sometimes it is the lowest of points in life that finally catapult us into action. I suppose this is basic human instinct, the determination to survive. But how amazing would it be if we didn't have to wait for these low points, and instead took action to prevent such drastic measures?

For Tosh and our family, one of the low points was during a week when Tosh had an exceptionally high fever. We were calling the doctor each hour to give a report on his health. He had been on one type of antibiotic that was not working, so the doctor gave him a new type. She said the new antibiotic would kick in within 12 hours, so we waited at home, watching the clock tick away as we anxiously awaited the effects of this superpower antibiotic to restore Tosh's health. But the exact opposite happened.

Around hour 10, Tosh started to walk across the living room to pick up a toy and collapsed. I had been so self-conscious about being an "overly paranoid" mom throughout the year of Tosh's health issues that I allowed myself to overlook how quickly Tosh was spiraling downward until he collapsed in front of me. I will never forget the look in Tosh's eyes as I drove him straight to the emergency room. It was as though the energy of life behind his eyes had disappeared. As I drove to the ER, my cheeks were flooded with tears. I felt, once again, helpless, and my fear for his life and the guilt of not bringing him to the hospital sooner consumed me. I kept asking myself what I'd been thinking, waiting so long. I would never be able to forgive myself if something terrible happened to him. The pressure of being a mom, and a new mom at that, is insurmountable.

Tosh survived that crisis, and he spent a few days in the hospital to allow the tissues to heal after the tonsillectomy. As days went by, Tosh's throat started to heal nicely, but he refused to drink water on his own (a common complication with young children after this procedure). The nurses suggested that we take Tosh for a walk down the halls to see if we could help him regain his thirst. Tosh had a great time walking and riding in the wagon on his return back to his room. We even saw an improvement in his mood, with a bit of laughter and smiles. But as we settled Tosh back into bed, alarms suddenly started going off from all of the monitoring machines.

It was just like you see in the movies. Tosh's heart rate plummeted, along with his oxygen levels. Eight doctors and nurses rushed into the room, scooped Tosh up, and swooped him away. The whole ordeal happened so quickly that I remember only bits and pieces of it. But the one thing that stands out crystal clear is a doctor asking me if I was okay. I thought for a moment and replied, "I think so." I was so grateful that support had arrived quickly to help Tosh. But when the doctor responded by saying, "Good, because we're headed to the ICU," I remember melting into a puddle, tears streaming down my face over the uncertainty of what lay ahead of us.

It is this uncertainty about our child's well-being that can push us to the breaking point. We may be uncertain of their physical survival. We may be uncertain if they will have to endure a life of medical complications. And we may be uncertain if our child will grow to feel confident socially and emotionally. In Tosh's first year of life, I doubted all of these things.

Sensory Condition Emerges

After spending four weeks at Primary Children's Hospital, we came home to an entirely new life. Tosh's physical symptoms were healing, but something new emerged: a sensory condition so severe that by the time he was two, a drop of water landing on his shirt would make him scream and try to tear his shirt off of his body. "It hurts, Mommy!" he'd sob.

We live in Jackson Hole, Wyoming, a cold and wintery place. At recess, Tosh wouldn't get dressed because the sensation of multiple layers of clothes on his skin was more than he could handle. He'd have massive meltdowns every morning as he tried to get dressed, without success. Eventually, we worked out that his clothes had to be soft sweatpants (with no cuffs at the bottom) and a soft shirt (tag removed) whose arms had to hit the perfect place on his wrist. He would only wear one type of sock, and it would take a solid 10 minutes or more just to get those socks on each morning. Now, imagine what getting ready for skiing looked like! It was nearly impossible. Every morning – every *day* – felt like an unbelievable struggle. Not only for Tosh, but also for my husband and me. We had to practice deep breathing, *a lot*. And there were plenty of times when our frustration and patience ran out, ending in yelling, which helped nobody and only left me with a knot of guilt and sadness. Tosh's behavior was not his fault. It was not because he wanted to make things difficult. My sweet boy had a sensory condition that we had not figured out.

There was yet another issue going on, which Tosh's teacher at the time fortunately recognized. Due to his chronic infections and health complications, Tosh suffered from impaired hearing the first couple years of his life – causing a speech delay. Luckily, we were able to qualify him to receive an IEP (Individualized Education Plan) through the special education department. This ensured that Tosh received support to help him manage his sensory issues and improve his speech. Knowing he had this support was *huge* for me, but my dream was to watch Tosh grow up feeling good in his body, rather than thinking he had to muscle his way through uncomfortable sensations on his skin and throughout his nervous system. Tosh felt like he lived in a body that wasn't "normal," and he felt isolated, believing that his experience was one other people had a difficult time understanding.

The Magic Answer

While all this had been going on with Tosh, my mom had been healing from chronic Lyme disease, which she'd suffered from for over twenty years. By working with an anti-inflammatory health coach and pushing inflammation from her body, the symptoms were literally melting away. I was impressed by her results, so I began investigating anti-inflammatory eating myself. Over the course of the previous 18 months, I had gained a ton of weight, and my energy was almost nonexistent. I was constantly bloated and nauseous, my hormones were totally out of whack, and I felt incredibly depressed. In fact, I did something I never thought I'd need to do: go on antidepressant medication. You see, I had always been the girl who *loved* everything in life and found the beauty in all situations, but watching my son suffer had shattered me, completely and utterly. After visiting several doctors to try to discover what was happening to my body, I was told that I was acquiring some sort of an auto-immune condition, but they couldn't figure out which one. I felt broken, alone, and scared, for myself and for my son.

But thanks to my mom's advice, (she has always forged the path toward health and healing), I began to work with an anti-inflammatory coach, and my symptoms began to reverse. The bloating and nausea disappeared. The weight melted off. My energy came back. The unexpected bonus was how darn good I felt mentally! It was a game changer. I no longer needed antidepressant meds because I felt *joy*, something that had been consistently missing from my life while Tosh was sick. Each morning,

I woke up and experienced what it felt like to have a clear mind. The brain fog lifted, and my memory improved. I was so much more efficient with my time, and my patience grew immensely. As good as it felt to heal physically, feeling good in my head far exceeded my expectations. It was this pot of gold that inspired me to keep going and stick with anti-inflammatory eating.

What I didn't yet know was that this practice of maintaining that way of eating would eventually save my life. (You can read more about my near-death experience due to parasites and Lyme along with the tale of healing in my first book, *Peace of Cake: The Secret to an Anti-Inflammatory Diet*.)

I had watched my mom heal from Lyme disease, my symptoms were reversing, and my dad also became inspired to follow this way of eating, which allowed him to get off of his high blood pressure medicine and decrease a calcium build-up in his heart. People all around me were healing from adopting and maintaining anti-inflammatory eating, so I was determined to try it with my son. If we could heal, so could he.

I set out on a two-week experiment, knowing that it typically takes 14 days for the body to fully process and eliminate all of the inflammation from the top inflammatory foods. I wanted to see how Tosh's body would respond once it was free of inflammation. Would it make a difference? And if so, how much?

The results were almost immediate and impressive. Within two weeks of following through with anti-inflammatory eating, Tosh's mood swings began stabilizing, his attention and focus started to improve, and I could see glimpses of him having more bandwidth to handle the heightened sensory conditions on his skin. The root of chronic conditions, including many behavioral issues, is linked to inflammation.[3] Take the inflammation out of the body, and the condition begins to improve! It's like a magic pill – but better, because it's natural and heals the root of the issues.

In those two weeks, I was 100 percent in integrity with what he ate. This meant that I packed carefully selected breakfast, lunch, and snacks for Tosh to bring to school. When he went to birthday parties or social functions, we made our own special treats (you can totally have cupcakes that taste delicious without the top inflammatory ingredients). I always made sure to have snacks packed in my bag and the car to ensure he never went hungry. It was a big priority for me to make sure Tosh never felt deprived or like he was on a diet. We were simply swapping out the inflammatory foods for foods that tasted similar but did not cause inflammation. Of course, we had to have a talk to begin this process (in Chapter 10, I'll share more with you about the most effective way to communicate with your child when adopting and maintaining anti-inflammatory eating), but as soon as Tosh and I discovered *his why* for trying this way of eating, he, too, was on board!

Within two months, Tosh's sensory condition had improved by 80 percent. He could put on socks in two minutes instead of ten. He still didn't like it if water got on his shirt, but he was no longer screaming and telling me it hurt. He was more grounded and a more engaged participant at school as his attention span increased. Because of this, his peers respected him, and he was able to make more friends. Tosh's confidence began to soar, and I discovered an entirely new version of my son, someone who now had the bandwidth to use coping skills to move through times when he was overloaded by sensory input. It was an incredible gift!

Due to a two-week science experiment, Tosh's life had greatly turned around, and so had ours as parents. Beyond the dramatic improvement of Tosh's sensory issues, he could now get a cold, and it would be just that – a cold. No longer was his immune system so compromised. No more crazy high fevers and visits to the hospital (or even doctors).

Tosh has been a healthy, thriving boy ever since. All of this gave us an incredible sense of relief as we observed Tosh improve each and every day. The mom-guilt began to dissipate because I felt empowered. I *did* have some control over helping Tosh feel better and gain increased good health. And I had control over my own health as well. What an incredible relief that was!

Chapter 3

The Secret Recipe

It All Begins with One Ingredient

When I started my anti-inflammatory eating journey, I learned the top inflammatory foods that wreak havoc on our health. These are the foods that I can confidently and definitively make a blanket statement about in regard to their ominous effect on inflammation in your body. These top inflammatory foods are processed sugar, processed wheat, cow dairy, refined oils, genetically modified foods (otherwise known as GMOs), and alcohol. Yes, I always save alcohol for the last, as I know that can be a tough one – though luckily not for our kids! (Juice, however, is just as bad – a kid's version of alcohol.) Of course, there are other inflammatory "foods" such as preservatives, additives, pesticides, *etc.* However, I find that when you eliminate the top six inflammatory foods and purchase organic fruits and vegetables, you pretty much eliminate all the other preservatives, pesticides, and chemicals that often hide in packaged food.

While there may be other foods potentially inflaming you (and those can vary from person to person), it's nearly impossible to identify them with certainty until you've removed the six big offenders that create chronic inflammation. When people come to me for a first health-coaching session, they will often carefully explain that they are sensitive to broccoli, carrots, and peas (just as an example), yet they're eating a diet packed full of processed sugar and inflammatory oils. Unless you are truly allergic to a food, meaning you have an allergic reaction that likely requires some form of medication to quickly reverse the symptoms, it is difficult to know what additional foods are absolutely inflaming you. With that said, it is very possible that peas could be inflaming you, and in order to find out, you want to remove these top major contributors of inflammation for at least two weeks *and then* see how your body responds to eating peas. One of the beautiful aspects of eating an anti-inflammatory diet is that food allergies often disappear over time. These allergies are often caused by a leaky gut (intestinal permeability where the lining of the small intestine becomes damaged, causing undigested food particles, toxic waste products, and bacteria to "leak" through the intestines and flood the blood stream), and anti-inflammatory eating has great success in helping to reverse that.

All too often I hear from people who have removed dairy and gluten from their diets (the most trendy forms of "clean eating"), yet they are still experiencing chronic symptoms. Now, I'm not dissing the removal of gluten and cow dairy. In fact, I'm all for it! However, there is one *huge* missing piece here, and that is processed sugar. Processed sugar is the number one inflammatory ingredient for kids (and tied with alcohol for adults). It is in *everything,* it seems, especially kid foods.

I recently took my little nephew grocery shopping to see if I could help him get excited about eating some different types of healthy foods. As we shopped our way through the baby/kid section, everything he pointed to that looked healthy was actually inundated with processed sugar. Worst of all was how healthy the packages made the food appear! There were beautiful, fresh, colorful pictures. The text said things like "all natural," "organic," or "sweetened with fruit juice" – yeah, fruit juice *concentrate,* which is one of the 50+ names for processed sugar. There is such a thing as organic junk food, and before I knew about anti-inflammatory eating, it was what I gave my son all of the time. And I felt really good about it! I actually thought I was doing a great job feeding Tosh healthy stuff.

How Is Inflammation Impacting Your Family?

I'm guessing that if your child is experiencing chronic symptoms, so are you, in some sort, shape, or size, even if it's just decreased energy. Chronic symptoms caused by chronic inflammation show up in many different ways. Inflammation targets the areas where we are most susceptible. This happens through genetic pre-disposition, over-use, or simply by targeting the vulnerable areas of the body. The most common symptoms people experience from chronic inflammation are low energy, poor sleep, inability to lose excess weight, digestive disorders, depression or anxiety, and aches and pains. What's important to remember is that *chronic* inflammation creates *chronic* symptoms. So if you are experiencing *chronic* discomfort, you can be sure that inflammation is a piece of the puzzle. While your symptoms may look different than your child's, the diagnosed conditions listed below may be within the range of what you experience. (Side note: this is not a complete list, but it will give you a sense of how inflammation can impact us.)

- Acne
- ADD/ADHD
- ALS
- Alzheimer's Disease
- Anxiety
- Arthritis
- Asthma
- Autism
- Autoimmune Disorders
- Bipolar Disorder
- Bloating
- Brain Fog
- Cancer
- Cardiovascular Disease
- Carpal Tunnel Syndrome
- Celiac Disease

- Chronic Headaches
- Chronic Muscle Pain
- Chronic Rash
- Crohn's Disease
- Cystic Fibrosis
- Dementia
- Depression
- Developmental Delays
- Diabetes
- Diverticulitis
- Eczema
- Epilepsy
- Fatigue
- Fibromyalgia
- Fibrosis
- Food Allergies
- GERD/Acid Reflux
- Graves' Disease
- Guillain-Barré
- Hair Loss
- Hashimoto's Disease
- Headaches
- Heart Attack
- Hepatitis
- High Blood Pressure
- High Cholesterol
- IBS
- Imbalanced Hormones
- Joint Pain/Stiffness
- Juvenile Diabetes
- Kidney Failure
- Lupus
- Lyme Disease

- Multiple Sclerosis
- Neuropathy
- Obesity
- Pancreatitis
- Parkinson's Disease
- Periodontitis
- Poor Memory
- Poor Sleep
- Psoriasis
- Seasonal Allergies
- Sensory Conditions
- Sinusitis
- Sleep Apnea
- Stroke
- Tuberculosis
- Ulcerative Colitis
- Ulcers

And the list just goes on and on....

This is why I refer to anti-inflammatory eating as the magic bullet. If we can remove the inflammation that is at the root of nearly all ailments, conditions, and diseases, we remove the reason for that condition to show up in the body. Inflammation is the one consistent player in all *chronic* symptoms. And while inflammation does not show up solely from what we eat (stress, lack of water, pathogens, and inactivity are also major contributors), diet tends to be the factor over which we have the most control to reverse or significantly improve many symptoms.

Scariest of all is that 1 in 10 children has asthma, 1 in 13 has food allergies, 1 in 10 has ADD, 1 in 6 has a developmental delay, 1 in 20 has epilepsy, and 1 in 68 has autism, with the numbers rising quickly. More than 23 percent of our youngest generation have juvenile diabetes, while heart disease is the fifth leading cause of death to children between 1 and 5 years of age. And, last but not least, cancer is the number one cause of death by illness in children, with more than 15,000 children diagnosed in 2014 alone.[4] Here in this book, you will gain the knowledge to push massive amounts of inflammation from your families' bodies. *We can save thousands of kids' lives with this information. We can heal even more. The question is, are you ready to close the gap between knowledge and action so you can move forward by "doing" rather than "knowing"?*

A Story of Regeneration

All of this healing is often possible without drugs and doctor visits. As you fuel your body with the food it is intended to eat, the cells that reside within actually begin to regenerate. It is a scientific fact that cells either regenerate or degenerate. There's no holding steady and staying the same. When we remove chronic inflammation, fuel the cells with real nutrition, provide enough water to the body, allow ourselves adequate rest, and move our muscles, the cells within our body magically begin to *regenerate.* This literally means you can grow young.

Suzanne, a recent client of mine, came to me with IBS-C, a form of Irritable Bowel Syndrome that causes constipation, extensive bloating, and exhaustion. She'd had this condition for over thirty years, since she was a teenager. Suzanne had been to loads of major medical universities and doctors, trying to find reprieve from her condition, but had only been given drugs that helped very little. While Suzanne considered herself a fairly good eater (no fast food restaurants for this girl), we discovered that many of the top inflammatory foods were embedded in her diet. When we first began working together, Suzanne would have a bowel movement around every five days (sometimes even longer). Remarkably, after only four weeks of eliminating these top inflammatory foods from her diet, she was going to the bathroom every other day. After six weeks, not only did her bowel movements become consistent on a daily basis but also her bloating went away and her energy soared!

When we have a chronic health condition, it's so easy to believe that "this is how it's always going to be." Our diagnosis can sometimes become our identity. But when we move from a state of acceptance and inactivity toward a state of healing, magic begins to unfold in all areas of our lives. Luckily for Suzanne, she believed in the power of healing and never gave up on finding an answer. In our last session, Suzanne told me, "I consistently feel so good. We don't even need to talk today! Anti-inflammatory eating has become super easy for me. I don't feel deprived, my energy is great, and there is no more bloating." For thirty years, the cells in Suzanne's body were degenerating, exacerbating her IBS-C symptoms, and *in six weeks we regenerated her cells and reversed her condition*. Want to join her in growing young in the next six weeks?

You're likely all ears for experiencing youthful health, but don't know how to take action without feeling entirely overwhelmed. My guess is that the idea of removing processed sugar, modern-day wheat, cow dairy, inflammatory oils, GMOs, and alcohol sounds far from easy to you. In fact, I bet it sounds downright overwhelming, not to mention depriving. I understand those emotions to the core. Trying to go out to eat and telling the server all that I cannot eat often felt like I was in a jail cell. Reminding myself of the top six inflammatory foods that I was to stay away from, especially at first, felt like a memory game in and of itself. But because I have walked my talk and eaten an anti-inflammatory diet for nearly a decade (not to mention coaching many beautiful clients as they shifted into a state of health through diet and lifestyle), I've been able to identify the number one biggest player creating most of the inflammation in your body right now.

The Key Player

Sugar is the Big Bad for sure. By removing processed sugar, the top inflammatory food, and swapping it out with something that tastes similar yet regenerates, rather than degenerates your cells, you can begin to lose weight, reverse adverse health conditions, raise your athletic game, experience a sensation of peace and grounded-ness, and experience high levels of joy in your life.

Processed sugar is a "food" labeled by the FDA a number of years ago as toxic, or so the story goes. Apparently as soon as this statement came out, the Big Sugar corporations launched a massive lawsuit disputing it – and won. Interestingly, when digging into all this, I found countless government-backed articles and "research" countering the idea that processed sugar is bad for us – but all of it was funded by the companies who had the most to gain from this misinformation: companies like Kraft, Coca Cola, General Mills, and Hershey Foods.

Consider this. Processed sugar is directly linked to type 1 and 2 diabetes, heart disease, tooth decay, cancer, fatty liver, and Alzheimer's, not to mention a slew of additional chronic health conditions. Yet the very doctors out there working to make our families healthier by encouraging us to reduce processed sugar intake actually worry about being shut down by the FDA because of the research they undertake and the results they find. Unfortunately, politics and deep-pocketed corporations still stand between the average American and the vital information that could reverse illness and even save lives.

Even for those of us who have educated ourselves about the health impact of processed sugar, it's still insanely hard to spot. That's because there are over fifty names for this highly inflammatory food, making it quite challenging for the consumer to avoid. It hides in everything! According to Dr. Robert Lustig (a pediatric endocrinologist at the University of California in San Francisco and a leading expert on the effects of sugar in human physiology), processed sugar is in 74 percent of the foods in every grocery store. While we all recognize sugar in cakes, cookies, and doughnuts, it's the hidden sugar that can get the best of us.

50+ NAMES FOR PROCESSED SUGAR

1. Barbados Sugar
2. Barley Malt
3. Beet Sugar
4. Brown Sugar
5. Buttered Syrup
6. Cane Juice
7. Cane Sugar

8. Caramel
9. Carob Syrup
10. Caster Sugar
11. Confectioner's Sugar
12. Corn Syrup
13. Corn Syrup Solids
14. Date Sugar
15. Dehydrated Cane Juice
16. Demerara Sugar
17. Dextran
18. Dextrose
19. Diastase
20. Diastatic Malt
21. Ethyl Maltol
22. Free-flowing Brown Sugars
23. Fructose
24. Fruit Juice Concentrate
25. Galactose
26. Glucose
27. Glucose Solids
28. Golden Sugar
29. Golden Syrup
30. Grape Sugar
31. High Fructose Corn Syrup
32. Honey (unless it's raw)
33. Icing Sugar
34. Invert Sugar
35. Lactose
36. Malt
37. Malt Syrup
38. Maltodextrin
39. Maltose
40. Mannitol

41. Molasses
42. Muscovado
43. Panocha
44. Powdered Sugar
45. Refiner's Syrup
46. (Brown) Rice Syrup
47. Sorbitol
48. Sorghum Syrup
49. Sucrose
50. Sugar (Granulated)
51. Treacle
52. Turbinado Sugar
53. Yellow Sugar

My challenge to you is to become a Renegade Researcher for the next two weeks. Read the label on every food you put into your mouth. If there is processed sugar in it, either opt out or swap it out for a food that uses *raw* honey, pure maple syrup, *raw* agave, liquid stevia, or unrefined coconut sugar. For the agave and honey, it's important that they be *raw*, meaning that they've never been heated or processed. Raw honey, in particular, has incredible anti-bacterial and anti-microbial properties. It is believed to help alleviate allergies and is full of vitamins and minerals. However, heating raw honey changes it on a molecular level and creates inflammation. The same is true of agave when it is processed. It is quite rare to find raw agave in packaged products, so be sure to keep your eyes peeled.

Beyond these concentrated sweeteners, it is important to know that whole fruit provides you with an array of vitamins, minerals, and antioxidants that support the healing of the body. As long as you are eating the *whole fruit*, rather than the fruit juice *concentrate*, the sugar you consume from items like bananas, oranges, apples, berries, pears, *etc.* has incredible potency to support living vibrantly.

If you're interested in knowing more about the direct correlation between health and the consumption of processed sugar, check out this timeline below. It demonstrates an indisputable connection between disease in the body and sugar consumption.

8,000 BC – Sugar cane is believed to be first domesticated in New Guinea. It spreads to China and beyond.

350 AD – Sugarcane growers in India discover and master how to crystallize sugar using a boiling process of refining cane juice.

11th Century to 1700 – Cane sugar is referred to as the white gold, costing upwards of today's equivalent of $50 per pound and making it unattainable for anyone other than the noble and rich.

1747 – Sugar beets are identified as a new source of commercial sugar, which drives down the price and makes sugar more affordable to the middle and lower classes. Because of the low cost, sugar is now added to candy, tea, coffee, and many other food items.

1800 – A French medical student identifies the first group of patients with rheumatoid arthritis, a condition in which the body's own immune system attacks the joint lining and cartilage. (Two centuries later, medical research will implicate sugar as a contributor to rheumatoid arthritis.)

1900 – The average British citizen now eats about 100 pounds of sugar per year, and the average American eats approximately 40 pounds a year.

1906 – A German physician, Dr. Alzheimer, first identifies a form of dementia. By the end of the 20th century, an estimated five million Americans will be diagnosed with Alzheimer's disease each year.

1910 – A medical explanation emerges in the US for the rising rates of diabetes: the pancreas of a diabetic patient was unable to produce insulin, a chemical the body uses to break down sugar.

1962 – An estimated 13 percent of American adults meet the criteria for obesity.

1967 – A Japanese scientist invents a cost-effective industrial process for using enzymes to convert glucose in cornstarch to fructose. High-fructose corn syrup derived from corn becomes a cheap alternative sweetener to beet and sugarcane sugar.

1975 – In the US, 400 new cases of cancer occur for every 100,000 people, or a total of 864,000 people each year.

1984 – Soft drinks companies such as Pepsi and Coca-Cola switch from sugar to the cheaper high-fructose corn syrup in US production facilities.

1992 – Cancer rates have climbed to 510 cases for every 100,000 people in the US.

2004 – Obesity now affects 24.5 percent of US adults.

2005 – Each US citizen now eats about 100 pounds of added sugars each year, up from approximately 40 pounds in 1900.

2008 – The average American eats 37.8 pounds of high-fructose corn syrup every year, mostly unknowingly because it is laced in thousands of processed food and drink products.

2008 – Obesity rates hit an all-time high of 32 percent for men and 35 percent for women. Obesity is considered a factor in nearly 400,000 deaths per year.

2011 – The United Nations declares that non-communicable diseases – diabetes, cancer, and chronic respiratory and cardiovascular disease – have overtaken infectious diseases as the world's leading cause of death.

2015 – The World Health Organization releases official guidelines on sugar intake. They recommend that free sugars (essentially sugars *other* than naturally occurring sugars in whole foods like fruit) make up no more than 10 percent of our daily diet, with a further suggestion to limit them to 5 percent. It is clear people in our modern world need new references and education around processed sugar, and The World Health Organization is beginning to step up to the plate at the conception of these new guidelines.[56]

If you Google this topic and dig a bit further, you will find loads of interesting information about the timing of the introduction of processed sugar and the negative effects of sugar intake. In addition, you will see the battle of medical professionals[7] against the FDA and Big Sugar corporations who have worked at trying to convince the general public that sugar is a nutritional component that should be added to everyone's diet as a way to keep one's weight in check.

Through work such as Dr. Robert Lustig's studies, sugar is beginning to be defined as a drug – as a poison connected to an array of health conditions causing death and overall suffering in life.

Someone could argue that it's not sugar creating such havoc in the general public's health. I agree that there are other contributing factors, such as dehydration, stress, lack of sleep, additional inflammatory foods, and environmental toxins. But facts are facts. Listen to Dr. Robert Lustig's keynote presentation *Sugar: The Bitter Truth.* Or even better, conduct a science experiment on yourself. Remove processed sugar (completely) from your diet for two to three weeks and listen to what *your body* has to say. You will come to find the truth. Processed sugar is frequently at the root of inflammation, and inflammation is at the root of nearly every chronic adverse health condition. Remove the sugar, and chronic symptoms begin to melt away.

So many of us don't realize how bad we feel! We might wake up with some nausea, but over time, it just becomes a pattern. Within a few months, that nausea is the new norm, and, a few months later, we don't remember what it felt like to wake up without nausea. The same is true of any chronic symptom. If it is low-grade and persistent, chronic illness becomes the new norm. Once they have adopted and maintained an anti-inflammatory diet, my clients very often tell me that they didn't realize they could feel this good. It is one of the greatest surprises in life, as Kevin Trudeau's famous quote states, "Most people have no idea how good their body is designed to feel." My challenge to you: Take that bold step, and allow yourself to feel all of the goodness by swapping out processed sugar.

In removing processed sugar from your diet, many of the top inflammatory foods will also fall to the wayside by default. This secret to eating an anti-inflammatory diet makes it so much more manageable. By removing processed sugar, you automatically eliminate 90+ percent of the alcohol, processed wheat, and cow dairy in your diet. In addition, you end up removing a significant amount of inflammatory oils and GMOs. It's my magic trick. Beyond magically eliminating many of these inflammatory foods by swapping out processed sugar for sweet treats that do not inflame, the removal of processed sugar alone has the power to heal many people's health conditions.

The key is to read those labels. Focus primarily on removing processed sugar and swapping it out with sugars that support your body. As you eat some of the tasty grocery store swaps in Part 2 of this book, make your own clean treats, or simply use the approved non-inflammatory sugars, all while drinking your water (more on that in Chapter 5), your body will begin to feel the best it has in years – possibly ever!

Heather, a sugar-holic, came to me asking for help. She told me that she simply could not continue living the way she was. She felt out of her mind and totally ungrounded. A mother of three young kids, she was constantly on the go, and while she had put forth worthy effort in the past, she could not figure out how to *maintain* anti-inflammatory eating. She had chronic knee pain, headaches, rashes, and anxiety. Life was not feeling amazing for Heather, and she had to do something about it. After following the steps in this book for two weeks, she said she no longer had a craving to indulge in a cocktail at the end of the day. After three weeks, her anxiety had significantly decreased. After five weeks, her knee pain had gone away, as well as her headaches. Her rashes significantly improved around this time as well. And within eight weeks, Heather felt confident that she would forever be able to maintain this way of eating that best supported her body. She no longer experienced sugar cravings! Heather felt grounded and in control of her life. She told me that she felt more comfortable in her own skin than she had ever remembered.

Join me as we forge new paths toward health and vibrancy. *And remember, the perfect time to start sometimes never arrives. All you have is now.* This very second could be the moment you make the decision to catapult your life forward in unimaginably beautiful ways.

The Clean-Eating Kid Tip

There are *so* many different clean and healthier brands of food using non-processed sugar these days. Take a few extra minutes the next time you're at the grocery store to investigate new foods. Even better, have your kids join you in reading the ingredients, and challenge them to find clean swaps for family favorites. It's a great practice for the whole family, and your kids will feel like they get to be in charge by finding new swaps. What kid doesn't love to be in charge?

Chapter 4

―――――

Be the Change
(in Your Child's Health)

Healing Starts with You

Whenever I talk to people about my line of work and the power anti-inflammatory eating can have on people, I often hear a comment like, "That sounds amazing! I know someone who could benefit from that." In life, it is *so much* easier to point our finger at others and suggest they step up to "the work" – whether that be through diet, exercise, mindfulness, or self-growth. As parents, we're wrapped around our kids' every move (especially if they are younger children), so it's very easy to see what needs to improve in their life, such as diet. And ... you're right! Chances are, they totally need to improve their diet. However, the success that your child will experience is *directly* related to your willingness to step up to the plate and adopt anti-inflammatory eating for yourself as well. While the name of this book is *The Clean-Eating Kid*, it is, in truth, written with the intent of helping your entire family overhaul their diet and therefore their health.

Here are some reasons your mind may tell you that this idea of your stepping up to the plate may not be necessary: "I already feel pretty good. I don't really have any issues." Look closely, now. Is this 100 percent true? The doctors may say you're healthy, but do you feel *vibrant*? If not, let's do a science experiment and see how vibrant you can feel! It's time to grow young. Another common thought is, "I don't have time to take care of myself *and* my child. Obviously he/she is most important, so I will put my effort there." True, we live in an increasingly busy world, and spare time seems nonexistent.

What would happen if I told you that you could increase your efficiency throughout the day by adopting and maintaining anti-inflammatory eating? What if you could actually create more time by having clearer and more grounded thoughts? Then would you be willing to give it a shot? When we adopt anti-inflammatory eating, our liver is freed up from burdensome toxins, which allows it to create more neurotransmitters sent directly to the brain. This very action allows for you to think more clearly, improves your memory, and you feel more grounded, which makes you more efficient with your time. Taking it a step further – and to likely the most important point: without you having your own good health, you will not be able to care for your child. As caregivers, it's *so* easy to put our kids first. Yet as caregivers, it's most important that we put ourselves first so that we can continue to take care of our children with our own physical vigor and clear minds.

Your Experience Will Guide the Way

When you walk your talk, you inspire others to hop on the clean-eating train, including each member of your family (and beyond).

My husband, Brock, has type 1 diabetes. When I was going through my 18-month anti-inflammatory certification and would come home from a training, I'd be so inspired by what I was learning and incredibly determined to help my husband heal, or at least significantly improve his symptoms. I wanted to tell him everything I had learned and why he needed to change his diet as soon as humanly possible. I was trying to *make* him change. I wanted it so darn bad for him, but he wasn't ready to make that commitment. The idea of changing his diet was overwhelming and intimidating. By my pushing and lecturing, I made things a million times worse as he rebelled by buying more candy, cinnamon rolls, and loads of processed foods. My heart sank, and I felt defeated.

It wasn't until I released the idea of Brock adopting anti-inflammatory eating that he came to and got more curious. His defense mechanism had dropped, as it does for all of us when we are no longer being pushed to do something. Brock watched my health transform. He watched Tosh's health transform, and he saw how inflammatory foods affected our daughter. Slowly but surely, Brock picked up pieces of anti-inflammatory eating, trying his own science experiments and feeling better on each step of the journey.

While our spouse's or significant other's experience is slightly different than those of our children, it's the same when it comes to us walking our talk first. When our family sees us feeling better, they begin to ask us about our process – which is much more powerful than us simply talking about it uninvited. Ultimately, they want to feel as good as we do. As they learn more, they will be inspired. This, my dear friend, is how you become the change you wish to see in your world.

So how does all of this work with helping your children adopt anti-inflammatory eating? In my experience, the more we feel how our personal body responds to inflammatory foods and, equally, how it feels when we *remove* inflammation from our body, the more we can help guide our children. If we do not experience the sensations and symptoms eating inflammatory foods brings about for ourselves, there is no way we can describe it to our children. No one wants to be forced to do something on their own, feeling singled out as if there is something wrong with them. However, kids love to feel a sense of belonging – in fact, it's so important that it is part of Maslow's Hierarchy of Needs.[8] According to Maslow, if you are unable to feel a sense of belonging, then positive self-esteem as well as self-actualization are theoretically unattainable. By adopting anti-inflammatory eating as a family (or at least with one parent participating), you can literally begin to shift your child's self-respect, self-esteem, status, recognition, strength, and sense of freedom. Ultimately, you help them to shape their desire to become the most that one can be.

Speaking of empowerment, when we give kids a choice, they feel respect and strength. Every kid wants to feel that way. So, during this process, it is absolutely key to help your child find *their why* for adopting anti-inflammatory eating, which could be totally different than *your why* for them. What matters is that they find a reason to try this science experiment of removing processed sugar from their diet for two weeks. We will talk more about how to communicate with your child to help them succeed with anti-inflammatory eating in Chapter 10. In the meantime, remember, our children are our teachers. While they may need delicious anti-inflammatory versions of treats like cookies, cakes, pizzas, and more to maintain this lifestyle, remember that you are likely the same. When we feel deprived, no matter our age, we will always tell ourselves *we deserve* a treat. But if we allow ourselves to eat *clean* treats, we no longer feel deprived. Anti-inflammatory eating becomes our way of life, not something we feel we need or deserve a break from.

The Clean-Eating Kid Tip

Throughout the rest of this book, you will find particularly important tips on how to bring your kid/s onto the clean-eating train without their feeling deprived and without you feeling overwhelmed. Remember, the more you step up and work the steps in each chapter yourself, the more your child will succeed. Once you have spent some time experiencing anti-inflammatory eating, you will be an expert at helping your child/ren do the same. You deserve to feel better, and so does our youngest generation … but they need your help.

Chapter 5

Start Removing Inflammation Without Changing Your Diet!

H₂O

How many of you have told yourself that you will start a diet right *after* your family vacation, *after* the Ben & Jerry's pint is empty, or *after* you make it through your next intense work week? You can fill in the words following *after* with any life obstacle, celebration, or event. That's where we create all of these rules about when and how change happens. Beyond the rules that we set for ourselves, it can be difficult to know where *your* entry point is for following an anti-inflammatory diet. Do you take sugar out of your diet first, or maybe dairy? Then again … the whole gluten-free thing is something worth looking into.

I have the perfect answer for you. It's perfect because it does not involve food, and you can begin right this very minute.

Drinking enough water is a key component in removing inflammation from your body. And it's perfect. You don't need to go to the grocery store or swap out foods to start, yet it makes the most profound difference. Even better, all you need is a water bottle or glass to begin – right here, right now.

I know you know about the importance of drinking water. In fact, everyone I have ever spoken to in regard to health knows the importance of hydration, yet very few people truly understand the critical role water plays in eliminating inflammation from the body. To be honest, if you walk away with nothing else from this book, promise me you will follow through with the single action step laid out in this chapter. Even if you do not change your diet, I can promise you that adding significant amounts of water to your day may be the single most powerful tool you can use on your journey to healing.

One of the first questions that I ask my clients during their initial consult is, "How much water do you drink?" The answer I most frequently get is, "Very little, but I'm just not thirsty." I love this answer because it opens up space for a very interesting science experiment, and science experiments are my favorite! I love them because it's one thing for someone to tell you what to do. It is entirely different when you allow your body to speak to you, and when you experience how your daily actions affect it. Truly, this is the gift I wish to bestow upon each and every one of you.

I have always been a big believer in explaining the *why* for doing something. So while you will experience your body speaking to you in our little science experiment, allow me to explain the *why* behind your not feeling thirsty, even when drinking a minimal amount of water. From an evolutionary standpoint, we have a thirst mechanism that can be turned on or shut off. When we were hunters and gatherers we would walk for hours, many times even for a day or two, moving from one water source to the next. Often there would be very little water available to drink during these migrations. In order to stop the physical discomfort thirst brings about, the thirst mechanism would be deactivated. This happened naturally whenever the body realized water was not available for it to drink. Instead of spending days feeling the suffering sensation thirst brings upon us, our body simply deactivates the thirst mechanism, a default response that continues unabated if we continue to drink little water. Likewise, if we start the morning drinking lots of water, it creates a signal saying a source of water is near us and available. This in turn activates your thirst mechanism, creating a sensation of more thirst as the amount of water you drink increases. This is your body's way of talking to you, saying, "Yes please! If water is available, I want *more* of it!" But don't take my word for it. Let me lay out a little science experiment for you to see how your body chooses to speak with you.

The body will ask for more water because so many of us have built-up toxins stored inside, and the only way to effectively get them out is through drinking enough water. Our bodies know this innately, which is why they will become thirsty, their way of asking for support to heal. And while it's true that drinking water brings on the dreaded extra bathroom breaks, it helps to do what I do. Get excited every time you have to pee! Remember – toxins are leaving your body each time. For all the things we can do to gain health, how amazing is it that simply peeing more often can begin to catapult us into vitality?

Ready for your first little science experiment, one that could indeed become the key action step that transforms your world? I know … sounds dramatic, but it's so true! Try it, and you can be the judge of my bold statement for yourself.

The goal of this experiment is to drink one gallon of water per day (for adults) and half to one ounce of water per pound of body weight for petite adults or children who have chronic inflammation. I know, that sounds like a staggering amount. Hang with me for one week, and then make your decision. What you will likely experience is a significant reduction in inflammation, the number on your scale dropping, less stiffness in your joints, a mental feeling of grounded-ness, and fewer cravings. Sound good? If so, here's the easiest way to accomplish drinking that gallon of water each day. If you try this with your child, follow the same steps while modifying the amount of water intake at each step.

The first thing you want to do is get a large water bottle, preferably one quart or 32 ounces. (You will be drinking four 32-ounce water bottles throughout the day or dividing the total number of ounces by four and drinking that amount in each water bottle.) When you wake up in the morning, go to the bathroom, weigh yourself (don't worry, it's fun because you can watch the inflammation melt off), and then chug the water bottle. For some, channeling their inner college-beer-drinking self helps bring them back to how easy chugging the water actually can be. If that was never you, no worries. Simply take your water and throw it down the hatch. The truth is, if you *focus* on drinking your water quickly and efficiently – in one sitting – you will make it happen. It only takes about 52 seconds to drink an entire quart of water if that is all you are doing.

The problem for most people is that they pour themselves a glass of water or a cup of tea/coffee in the morning. They begin to check emails and Facebook, pack their kids' lunches, and get dressed. Halfway through their water (if they are lucky enough to get themselves a glass of water before the coffee and tea), it's time to leave for the day. Because of all the distractions, their water was never drunk, or at least not much of it. This automatically sends a message to the body, telling it to keep the thirst mechanism low – not much water is available today.

If instead, you stand in one place and drink your quart of water *before* you do anything else other than use the restroom and weigh yourself, your body thinks you have a huge source of water available to you, and you actually become thirstier the more water you drink. It's such a fun experiment! Once you have the morning chug down, you will want to immediately fill up your water bottle again.

Have you ever been thirsty with an empty cup sitting right in front of you, but while you wanted to drink, you didn't because of the effort required to get up and fill up your glass? If you're like 99 percent of us, the answer is yes. So let's avoid that happening by filling up your water bottle right away.

The next goal is to drink your second quart of water by lunch. Ideally, you drink water from your second water bottle between breakfast and lunch. Around noon, or when you stop for lunch, the idea is to chug any water left from water bottle two. Repeat for water bottle number three, chugging any remnants at 3 in the afternoon, with the last water bottle going down the hatch by 6 pm. I encourage finishing off your last quart of water by 6 pm (likely close to your dinnertime) so that you have time to use the bathroom often enough before going to bed. That way you won't wake up as frequently to use the bathroom at night.

Speaking of the bathroom … I know what you're thinking. "I'm going to have to pee every two seconds!" Truth be told, you will have to pee quite a bit the first couple of weeks that you implement this science experiment. The reason is that you are pushing crazy amounts of inflammation (or toxins) out of your body and into your bladder. Imagine your bladder as if it were an empty pond. As the inflammation and toxins are pushed out of your body, they condense in your bladder. As you can imagine, sitting in a pool of toxins is no fun, so the bladder sends a signal to your brain sharing the need to eliminate the condensed toxins ASAP. What you will find is that you will frequently need to pee, but the elimination will likely be quite short. This is because, while there may not be a ton of fluid in your bladder once it signals the need to eliminate, there are a ton of toxins. As you continue with your consistent water drinking, you will find that the built-up chronic inflammation begins to disperse, lowering the concentration of toxins in your bladder and allowing your body to hydrate as it is meant to. How does this help you? Within a few weeks of time, you will be peeing much less often, and your elimination will be more thorough and take time. This is a good sign that significant inflammation has left your body!

Why is all of this water drinking so important? Peeing and sweating are the two major ways people eliminate inflammation from their bodies. There are other methods, but these are the simplest, most efficient ways to eliminate inflammation. And while we cannot sweat all day long, we can drink water and pee all day long. Water is to your liver and kidneys what gasoline is to a car. If your car is running on empty, or if it has poor-quality gasoline going in, it will slowly sputter down the road. However, if your car is on full and has high-quality gasoline, you will have no problem zipping down the road to your desired destination. The same is true of water. If you drink enough clean water (one gallon per day for the purpose of eliminating inflammation from the body), your liver will have superpower abilities to process the built-up toxins and inflammation residing within you that can cause a host of major issues if not flushed out.

If the liver and kidney do not have enough clean water, they cannot process all of the toxins being added to the body, so toxins are reabsorbed. From here, one of two things happens. Option one: the toxins are directly reabsorbed back into your organs. When this happens, you can become quite ill, quickly. The second possibility is that the body will create a storage space for these toxins by pushing them as far away from the organs as possible in pockets of fat tissues. If there is a large overload of toxins being reabsorbed in the body, you will experience an increase in body fat because the body is literally creating more fat to store the toxins in. It is a survival mechanism to push the toxins as far away from the organs as possible.

It's important to note that many of my clients lose 2–10 pounds in the first week of working with me (even if they're not really looking to drop weight), simply because they are finally fueling their liver through water consumption, which allows toxins and inflammation to be pushed out of their body. I absolutely love watching this transformation take place. Not only does the number on the scale typically decrease, but people start to notice how much better they feel. One of the top benefits of increasing water intake to a gallon per day is the exponential increase in energy that people experience. Along with that increase in energy, people will often find that their digestion begins to work more smoothly, their joints have more mobility, their skin clears up, and they sleep better at night. In fact, one of my clients just recently wrote to me saying that after one week of drinking a gallon of water per day, her gut is finally working and regularity has come back for the first time in months. All of this simply by increasing the amount of water consumed. Pretty cool, right?

Some people question the amount of water I encourage them to drink. There is a lot of debate in the nutritional world about this topic. Some organizations recommend you drink eight glasses of water per day, while opposing views say that's not enough. And then again, others simply say drink when you're thirsty (tricky to do if the thirst mechanism is shut off). Needless to say, all of those organizations are looking at water intake in terms of hydration. We are looking at it to both hydrate and upregulate the detox pathways (essentially, to push out toxins as easily and effectively as possible.)

Imagine your body as a dried-out riverbed filled with rocks and pebbles, each representing the toxins and inflammation trapped in your cells and organs. Now let's imagine a slow and steady trickle of water beginning to run down the riverbed. The water will push out *some* sand and small pebbles, but we are looking to push out large quantities of stones and boulders. The goal is not to simply stay alive by eliminating small amounts of inflammation, but to thrive by getting rid of the smoldering chronic inflammation. So now imagine a torrential downpour; the riverbed fills up entirely. Soon the pebbles, stones, and boulders are pushed downstream and out of the riverbed. This is the same concept for your body. It's one thing to be hydrated; it's a whole new level to use the consumption of clean water as a tool to eliminate inflammation from your body.

So while the peeing may be obnoxious for a few days, think of pivoting your thoughts ever so slightly. Instead of predetermining that they are an annoyance, remember that peeing and sweating are the two primary methods for eliminating both inflammation and fat from the body. So embrace the peeing. Know that through this simple step, you are making tremendous headway in gaining health and eliminating inflammation from your body.

Now go find yourself a quart of water, and give it a good chug.

Juice

I simply cannot end this chapter without mentioning the negative effects of juice on your child's health. As I mentioned earlier in this book, alcohol ties with processed sugar as the number one inflammatory food a person can put into their body. Juice is to a kid what alcohol is to an adult.

It seems that nowadays, children are given sippy cups full of juice rather than water. When your child says he is thirsty, how often do you offer water before you give him milk or juice? And has juice become so habitual that even if you do offer up water, he craves a nice hit of processed sugar (*also known as juice concentrate*) to satisfy his taste buds and cravings?

Ninety-nine percent of all juice is made from juice concentrate, which means it is processed sugar: the number one inflammatory thing you can give him. That means he's ingesting a toxin – often on a daily and sometimes even an hourly basis! And if processed sugar is the number one most inflammatory food we can put into our body – imagine the compounding effect.

So what to do about juice? If you cut it down with water, does it solve the problem? Not really. Cutting it down does eliminate the amount of processed sugar, but that's like saying it's okay to drink ¼ teaspoon of bleach in your coffee instead of ½ teaspoon. Either way, it's toxic and is going to make you sick. But what you can do is look for fresh-squeezed juice or juice that is not made from concentrate. My family always buys fresh-squeezed juice from the store, and I never give it to my kids without them first drinking a glass of water. I want them to know that the fresh-squeezed juice, while it is a liquid, cannot replace water. Instead, it is a beautiful treat loaded with vitamins. There are a few brands and specific flavors of juice that are not made from concentrate. You can find them in the grocery store swaps in the back of this book. Even better: swap out juice for coconut water! My daughter loves coconut water, which has immeasurable health benefits for anyone who drinks it.

The Clean-Eating Kid Tip

For hydration purposes alone, people are encouraged to drink a half-ounce of water for every pound of their body weight. So if you have a child who weighs 50 pounds, the minimum amount of water they should drink is 25 ounces *to stay hydrated*. If your child has a chronic condition due to inflammation, then encouraging even a bit more water is an excellent way for him/her to feel better more quickly. Use your creativity to find ways to make drinking water fun and habitual.

For example, both of my kids always drink a 10-ounce glass of water before they go to school (to let their body know water is available). I ensure they have water bottles at school each day and remind them to drink it with a specific goal, such as, "See if you can drink one *whole* water bottle today at school so that you can feel strong and focused." (Substitute the specific goal your child is looking to accomplish by changing their diet. See more about this in Chapter 7.)

My kids particularly love drinking water out of fun and colorful straws or cups. Sometimes we have water-chugging competitions at home with the whole family, which always brings about extra giggles. And last but not least: help your child create a habit around drinking water. For example, we have created a habit in our family to drink water every time we get in the car. A few additional ideas are to create a routine of drinking water right before the kids leave for the bus, eat a meal, play a sport … you get the idea. The more they practice drinking water, the more natural it will become. Just like it will for you!

Chapter 6

Sugar: It Makes a Difference

*We now know that food is medicine, perhaps the most powerful drug
on the planet with the power to cause or cure most disease.*
— Dr. Mark Hyman, MD

How to Swap out the Inflammatory Sugars for Sugars that Improve Health

Sugar has a bad rap in general when it comes to diet and nutrition. There are sugar detox programs, sugar avoidance counselors, and different theories that address whether or not sugar should be removed from the diet. To simplify the confusion, all of the advice I am giving you is specifically designed to remove inflammation from your body. With that said, here's what you need to know.

Not all sugar is bad. And when we begin to remove all sugar from our diet, we can feel incredibly deprived. Not to mention that we may miss out on key nutritional components such as antioxidants, minerals, and vitamins if we avoid whole fruits.

There is often confusion about what constitutes a "no sugar" diet. Sometimes that means eating no sugar of any kind, including naturally occurring sugar. For the sake of this book and for the sake of removing inflammation from your body, it's important to remember that the sugar from whole fruit is not inflammatory. If you chose to work with an anti-inflammatory health coach, they may suggest certain types of fruits, but it all depends on your individual goal.

Rather than memorizing all 50+ names of processed sugar in order to avoid them, I find it easier to focus on the types of sugars that work well for our body. There are five main non-inflammatory sugars that I use. The first is raw, organic honey. It's important that it's raw, because heating honey changes the molecular make-up and creates an inflammatory response. My second favorite sugar swap is *pure organic maple syrup*. I'm talking Vermont-style maple syrup, not Aunt Jemima's imitation maple syrup. Grade B is actually the best because it's the least refined version and, as a bonus, costs less. My third swap is whole fruits. If you're looking for something to eat that is super convenient, really fast, and extra tasty, then grab yourself a banana, apple, pear, some berries, or another fruit of your liking.

If you experience a major craving for sweets or want a delicious sweetener for baked goods, pick yourself up some Medjool dates. They are nature's natural form of caramel, and the best sugar swap in muffins, pies, cookies, and cakes. Unrefined coconut sugar is my fourth sugar swap. While it is a bit more processed, it doesn't typically inflame people and has a very low glycemic rating. For my last swap, I like to use liquid stevia. I prefer stevia in the liquid form because it is less refined and better for you. In fact, recent research shows that it has anti-bacterial properties – a fun fact for you! There are zero calories and zero sugar grams in it. Also, and this is important to note, liquid stevia is very sweet in taste. So you can add just three to five drops to a cup of coffee or tea and have a nice, sweet taste to replace the sugar that you might have put in your coffee before reading this book.

There's another type of sugar I'm often asked about as a good sugar alternative: agave. Agave has a great reputation in the health industry, but it's a little bit tricky. Similar to honey – only more intense – agave is usually found in its processed version, and, like honey, has been changed molecularly so that it creates an inflammatory response in the body. This response is not nearly as severe as those 50+ inflammatory sugars I told you about, but it's one that I recommend staying away from most of the time unless it is raw. If you can find raw agave, it's a lovely substitution for processed sugar as well. It is, however, a bit more challenging to find in any sort of commercial items or packaged foods.

Why is it so important to remove processed sugar from our diet when trying to eliminate the chronic inflammation in our body? Processed sugar is the number one inflammatory food, along with alcohol. Processed sugar has been deemed more addictive than cocaine through thermal brain scans that were conducted by the aforementioned Dr. Robert Lustig. Processed sugar has been directly correlated to a host of conditions and diseases such as cancer, autoimmune disorders, thyroid and hormone dysfunction, skin conditions, depression, anxiety, obesity, lower metabolism, heart disease, leaky gut … truly, the list goes on and on. Remember that inflammation can show up differently in each person, because it targets the areas where you're most susceptible. So sugar will also affect each person differently. It will target those weaker, more susceptible areas in your body and will make underlying conditions more pronounced. It is truly your body's way of speaking to you.

When your knees hurt, when a rash breaks out, when your stomach is upset, when you have a chronic pounding headache, when your hormones are out of whack, or when you're feeling depressed, your body might be telling you that whatever you're giving it is not the right recipe for what it needs to succeed and to thrive. You are meant to feel your very best. I'm here to help that become your reality.

So let's talk a little bit about the idea of removing processed sugar from your body and from your diet. My guess is that if you've never done this before, you're feeling a certain amount of anxiety tugging at your heart and stomach. (Your kids will feel the same way too.) Many times when I've conducted workshops and challenged people to swap out processed sugar for a week, there is an immediate sense of panic that overcomes each participant. True to how I live life, I always bring some sort of clean treat from one of the recipes in *Peace Of Cake*, or a grocery store swap from the back of this book. What I hear time and time again is, "Oh, my gosh, I had no idea clean eating could taste so good!" Finding anti-inflammatory treats to have on hand as you remove processed sugar from your diet is one of the most important things you can do to set you and your family up for success.

Some processed sugar is easy to spot: cupcakes, cookies, cinnamon rolls, alcohol. These are foods that you know, even without reading the ingredients, are going to have processed sugar in them – unless, of course, you're making a special food swap using non-inflammatory sugars.

As a Renegade Researcher, your goal is to begin reading the *ingredients label.* Not the nutritional fact label that tells you how many grams of sugar or grams of carbs or grams of protein are in the product, *but rather the types of ingredients that are in the product.* The reason we focus on this is because you have choices. You could eat a banana, which has naturally occurring fruit and lots of fiber, and it could have 15 grams of sugar in it. Likewise, you could pick up a granola bar that has 15 grams of sugar, but that sugar comes directly from cane sugar, high-fructose corn syrup, or one of the top inflammatory sugars. One food, the banana, is going to support your health. The other food, the granola bar, contains the sugar that will degenerate the cells in your body and will cause high levels of inflammation.

My challenge to you: Begin swapping out processed sugars right away – even starting today (for yourself … we still have some talking to do before we introduce it to the kids). Read every single ingredient label of every single food that goes into your mouth, because education is power. And you are here to become empowered, to gain good health, and to alleviate all of those chronic symptoms that have been bugging you for months or years, so that you can feel and live the life you're meant to live of radiant health, vibrant energy, and joy.

If you read the ingredients on Earth's Best Apple Granola bars, you'll find three different names of inflammatory sugars: organic cane syrup, organic rice syrup, and organic apple juice concentrate. Of course there are additional inflammatory ingredients on the ingredient list, but based on this process of swapping out processed sugar, you would not eat this bar and therefore would avoid the additional top inflammatory ingredients, including a number of wheats, organic butter flavor, canola oil, and multiple preservatives. Instead, you could swap this out for an Apple Pie Lara Bar or a Cinnamon Apple RX bar (you'll find grocery store swaps in Part 2 of this book).

I call that first type of granola bars "organic junk food." The food industry tricks us constantly with their labeling and with their marketing into believing that we're putting healthy nutrition into our bodies, when instead, while there may be some healthy ingredients, we are eating added inflammatory foods that counteract any health benefit we might receive.

In order to get the best bang for your buck, you don't have to remove all sugar, only the processed versions. You truly can have your cake and eat it too! What is important is that you give yourself foods whose sugars do not cause an inflammatory response. Give yourself abundance rather than deprivation. As you move forward, tell yourself that you can have anything you want. You can make cookies and treats and snacks. Whatever you can imagine, you can make it or find it with non-inflammatory ingredients. It is this shift, this food swap, that will raise you up to a level of health you may have never before experienced. More importantly, these food swaps, along with thinking thoughts of abundance rather than depletion, will allow you to continue eating this way for a lifetime. Our goal is to avoid diet mentality. This is not a "when I lose 10 pounds, I'll go back to eating the same way" program. Because when you lose 10 pounds and go back to eating the same way, you'll just gain another 10 pounds, and the chronic inflammation will continue to show up in an array of different symptoms.

This is not a calories in, calories out type of diet either. Always remember, *what* you're putting into your body matters more than *how much* you put into your body. If you are hungry, fuel yourself, and if you are full, allow your body the time and space to digest what you ate.

Our Kids Deserve Sugar, in "Moderation"?

It is our society's general belief that everything can be good for us in moderation. And even more so, I have found a common belief that children "deserve" to eat sugar. I believe in everything in moderation, at least when it comes to foods that support our health. For example, I will eat non-inflammatory sugars such as pure maple syrup or raw honey in moderation. I don't eat large amounts of it, but I have it for special occasions, or sweet treats. This is where I believe the original statement of "everything in moderation" came from: eating a variety of the whole, natural foods that we were meant to eat.

The problem is that our societal beliefs around dietary moderation have been shaped by the food industry. Why would we want to put a toxin (in any amount) into our children's bodies in the belief that they deserve it? Sugar is hidden in everything, and because of this, we continue to eat more and more of it. The more sugar we eat "in moderation," the sicker our youth continue to get. It's time to put a stop to even the smallest amount of toxic sugar intake so we can put our bodies into a state of healing.

Once, I was as deluded about this as anybody. I looked around at people who ate sugar on a daily basis, even if only the stuff that was hidden in processed foods, and felt that if they could be healthy while eating those foods, then this whole sugar hype must have been blown way out of proportion. There were so many people eating processed sugar each day who appeared healthy, so sugar must not be the culprit – or so I thought.

I believed it was a narrow population that was negatively impacted by processed sugar. But the years I've been coaching have dispelled that myth. As soon as I tell people that I am an anti-inflammatory health coach, they immediately start telling me about the ailments affecting them. I kid you not: 99 percent of the people I randomly introduce myself to as an anti-inflammatory health coach tell me about the chronic symptoms they experience, and those symptoms all have inflammation at their root. These are not just my clients, but people I meet at the grocery store, in the post office, or at social engagements. Many of these people appear to be healthy on the outside, but appearances can be deceiving. It is the chronic toll of symptoms showing up on the inside that is so insidious. The truth is, those people who supposedly ate sugar and were never affected by it were in actuality a false story I told myself. Most, if not all, of those people were struggling with their own symptoms, yet I had created a story to convince myself that nothing was wrong with their bodies.

This is natural. As humans, we judge and create stories. In fact, this is so prevalent that a large portion of my work is dedicated to helping people experience the connection between food and the symptoms that they have so they can get out of the stories and align with *truth*.

The reality is that the processed sugar we consume each day is scientifically shown to cause inflammation. Period. It is not a theory, or an idea formed by a bunch of hippies. It is *truth*. It is science.[9] As stated by Dr. Frank Hu, professor of nutrition at Harvard Health, "The effects of added sugar intake are higher blood pressure, inflammation, weight gain, diabetes, and fatty liver disease — are all linked to an increased risk for heart attack and stroke."

Because most people consume significant quantities of processed sugar, the inflammation stacks up to become more than the body can handle over time. As you can see by the timeline in Chapter 3, the increased consumption of processed sugar directly correlates with the increase in chronic conditions throughout society, yet we continue to put it into our bodies. It's not for a lack of knowledge (for most people), but rather a psychological and even physiological dependence. Sugar is addictive, tasty, and convenient. In fact, a study out of Bordeaux, France, demonstrated that processed sugar is actually *more* addictive than the drug cocaine.[10] And while this addiction is real, it's complicated by our food industry.

What's happening in our bodies? Quite simply, the sweet taste of sugar releases feel-good hormones that give us a temporary feeling of pleasure. Sadly, this pleasure response doesn't last long – and the waning pleasure quickly creates a desire for the next "hit." The more we load our body with sugar, the more we crave it. But there's more to this addictive cycle. More times than not, when we are: tired, stressed, or hungry (chronic states of being in this modern-day era), we reach for foods to comfort us. And for many, that comfort comes in the form of processed sugar.

So now, take a step back, and look at the big picture.

1. When we are tired, stressed, and hungry, we tend to reach for processed sugar.
2. As soon as we eat the sweet stuff to alleviate fatigue, stress, or hunger, a chemical reaction takes place in our body that creates a temporary sense of relief.
3. This relief tappers off quickly, leaving us even more stressed, so we reach for more food.
4. Whereupon the chemical response again takes place, and this cycle continues.

To make matters worse, food companies are constantly labeling their foods, "natural," "heart healthy," "organic," "gluten-free," "vegan," and more, making us think we are making good choices when in fact processed sugar still lurks in the ingredients list. We think we are eating healthy, and don't understand why we don't feel well. This is why we must become renegade researchers to take back our health.

That's a lot to overcome. So if you're just beginning to eat an anti-inflammatory diet and are experimenting with swapping out processed sugar, remind yourself that you're on a journey. No one is perfect. If you've fallen off the bandwagon and are trying to get back on, remember we all "fail" at times.

When your family joins you, the trial and error process becomes even more pertinent. It took me two years to get to a place where Tosh was eating a complete anti-inflammatory diet. He stayed with it for over three years, but just this week, he fell off the wagon (in a major way). Tosh ate more inflammatory foods this past week than he had in an entire year or more. I don't know why it happened exactly. The perfect storm happened, and I decided to go with the flow so Tosh could really feel the contrast his body experiences when eating clean versus not. It was a great learning opportunity for him, and a tough lesson. But Tosh's body made clear to him the importance of clean eating if he wants to feel well.

The truth is, there is no such thing as failure, as long as you learn from your experience. In fact, I secretly get really excited when a client falls off the bandwagon, as they then have the gift of experiencing the contrast of feeling great and then not so great. Feeling unwell after eating processed sugar (or a food that does not serve your body) is simply your body speaking to you, asking you not to eat or drink that again. It's a beautiful opportunity to learn about you and what makes you feel good. If you choose to consciously look at your experience through this lens, you will gain so much.

The idea is to keep walking toward an objective of eliminating processed sugar from your diet while eating the sugars that do not inflame you. The ultimate goal is to eat only those foods that support you rather than those that cause degeneration. With that said, we are human and perfectly imperfect. With each forward step you take, remember to celebrate all accomplishments, big and small. If you fall off the wagon and eat a piece of cake, the power is in hopping right back on the clean-eating train. Drink your water, eat some clean protein, and prepare your food ahead of time so success is more likely in the week ahead of you. (Look for more tips to hop back on the clean-eating train, to detox, and to stop cravings in their tracks in Chapter 8.)

When looking to eliminate inflammation from your body, the ultimate goal is to remove all processed sugar rather than to eat it in moderation. But notice, I said *ultimate.* There are two subtle ways of thinking that end in radically different scenarios. If you believe that the ultimate goal is to eat everything in moderation, and if you already have chronic inflammation stacking up in your body, then processed sugar, in moderation, could be the culprit not allowing your body to completely heal. On the other hand, if you believe that the ultimate goal *is* to swap out all processed sugar, but you are human so you fall off the wagon from time to time, yet continue to take strides forward, the healing in your body will become inevitable and the inflammation will eventually fall off of you. Ultimately, an improvement is an improvement, and that is what we continue to strive for. As author and pastor Naeem Callaway says, "Sometimes the smallest step in the right direction ends up being the biggest step of your life. Tiptoe if you must, but take the step."

Everyone has a different journey, and everyone has a different process when it comes to clean eating. With that said, clients often share in their first session with me that they eat really well, so they are confused about why they don't feel better. They typically say something like this:

"I eat a mostly healthy diet. It's pretty clean, and I exercise and take good care of myself. I can't understand why my arthritis won't go away, or why my digestive issues are so insistent. I have headaches a couple of times each week, and I feel like I'm depressed. I have really low energy. I know this is coming from inflammation, but I really do eat so well."

The truth is that the food industry and society have created a norm for eating "healthy" that in reality often creates chronic inflammation. Again, it is all perspective. When we can see the truth of how our bodies respond to the foods and drinks we consume, then we are no longer vulnerable to what others say or how great the latest food marketing scheme seems. You can't fight reality. Actually, you can, but trust me … it traps you in a never-ending vicious cycle until you are ready to own up to your truth.

Sarah came to me suffering from debilitating chronic symptoms that were hampering her on a daily basis. She was a mom of two young children, owned her own business, and had an amazing life. The problem was that she was so sick, she could no longer live that life. Sarah would go to bed at 4:30 in the afternoon, unable to spend time after school with her children. She had to cut her work hours down to seven hours per week. She could not commit to social engagements with her friends, as she did not know if she would be in bed or able to attend the event. She longed to be able to pick up the athletic endeavors that had brought her much joy, but she was too ill. Sarah felt hopeless. She had tried the Paleo Diet, been to every doctor in the region, and was seeking out-of-town specialists when we began working together.

As Sarah became a Renegade Researcher, she followed this process and *truly listened to her body.* Sarah was able to learn what caused inflammation by *feeling* and *listening* to her body every time she ate and drank. Within six weeks of swapping out inflammatory foods for those that do not inflame, Sarah was swimming laps at the pool, reading to her kids at night, and following her dreams of becoming a successful entrepreneur. It was amazing to see how Sarah's inflammation had been impacting her relationships, her career, and her ability to have fun exercising. She got her life back. You can do that too. In fact, your entire family is about to step into the transformation of their lives.

The Clean-Eating Kid Tip

Notice how often you fall prey to the belief that your child deserves inflammatory foods. There is no judgment here – I, too, can fall prey to this idea. It's especially easy to fall for this, since our society tends to equate inflammatory foods with rewards. When I heighten the awareness around my own thoughts on this topic, I begin to see how easily every single day could be a celebration and a reason to eat inflammatory food.

Reframing our thinking around what a reward is and how to participate in celebrations without causing harm to the body at the same time is an incredible practice. To begin with, food swapping is an easy solution, as is giving gifts or, even better, quality time spent with mom and dad. Quality time does *not* have to involve getting an ice cream cone together. Instead, it could mean playing in the park together, going for a walk, or swimming at the pool.

I encourage you to simply begin noticing how often you bend the rules (for yourself and your kids), and where healthier food options could be substituted. When dealing with a chronic health condition, closing the gap that lies between mostly eating healthy to eating healthy nearly all the time can be the difference between regeneration and degeneration.

Chapter 7

How to Get Your Child on the Clean-Eating Train (and Keep Them There)

Find Their *WHY*, Beyond Yours

Take a moment to think about your child's symptoms. Maybe they do not have a chronic condition, and simply want to get big and strong. Maybe they've been diagnosed with an illness, experience chronic symptoms, or struggle behaviorally. Let's pretend your child has a sensory condition (just insert any chronic symptoms he/she is experiencing in place of the ones I'll mention). For a child with a sensory condition, putting on socks can feel incredibly painful to him. And when he finally gets his socks on, the seam and tag on the inside of his pants makes him want to crawl out of his skin. He gets to school, where he is required to put on his gym shoes, but the laces are either too tight or too loose. I think you get the drift here. This child is consumed by thinking about how his skin feels and is unable to focus on what he's supposed to be doing at school.

He is now asked to sit down and follow the reading or math lesson, but all he can think about is how uncomfortable he feels in his body. He wants to do well and get approval from teachers and peers, but his mind is distracted by every sensation: his shoes seem too tight, his pants are rubbing in different places along his legs, and the tag in his shirt feels like a knife rubbing into his neck.

Subconsciously or not, this child is having to work through the physical discomfort of his chronic symptoms and the mental and emotional impact of not being able to control it. He may experience repercussions as a consequence, such as getting in trouble for not paying attention in school, being made fun of by his peers, or experiencing frustration from other adults. That's a lot for anyone, much less a child, to work through at any given moment.

Now let's see how your child's condition is affecting *you*. In our hypothetical example, just getting your child ready for school, or ready to head out the door, takes tremendous effort. Talking him through coping skills to deal with the sensation of the socks on his skin takes time and patience. And, just like in school, where he is preoccupied by trying to deal with the uncomfortable sensations on his skin, he likely isn't able to pay attention to the directions you are giving him about packing his backpack, brushing his teeth, or completing unfinished homework. All of this is happening at the same time you are trying to get yourself ready for the day. All of the sudden, your morning is looking to be chaotic, frustrating, and stressful – none of which are good for you or your child.

Thinking about the above or your own situation, it's easy to see *your why* for your child to adopt anti-inflammatory eating. You probably want your mornings to go more smoothly (I know I certainly did, which in my case I knew would happen if Tosh's sensory conditions improved). But *your child's why* will likely be because he wants to make more friends or be able to get dressed and out to recess quickly so he has more time to play, for example. Again, this will happen if his sensory conditions improve. But what will motivate him to cooperate with a two-week science experiment and see what happens when he follows anti-inflammatory eating is different from your motivation. It is *his why.*

Take a moment to think about how completely your child's symptoms are affecting him and getting in the way of his living the day-to-day life he dreams of. This is an important step to help you discuss *his why*, which will help you get his buy-in to try a two-week science experiment.

Give Your Child a Job

If we want our kids to adopt this way of eating, we need to give them a role or a job within the family specific to anti-inflammatory eating. When I work with families, I always assign kids the role of Renegade Researcher. We humans – and especially children – love to feel in control. As the Renegade Researcher, your child gets to screen all of the food your family buys and eats for processed sugar. If the ingredients list comes up inflammatory, then they get to go on a treasure hunt through the store (or in the back of this book) to find similar options without inflammatory ingredients. This practice has dual benefits. The first is to ensure that your kids feel like anti-inflammatory eating is being done *with them*, rather than *to them*. The second is to give them ownership and make the process fun. It's one of the easiest ways to get your kids invested in living a new lifestyle.

Supply a Variety of Tasty, Clean Treats for Your Family

Can you think of a time when you followed a diet and felt deprived, yet stuck with it as a lasting lifestyle? I'm guessing the answer is no, because any time we feel deprived, there is a deep desire to comfort the deprivation. This applies to all aspects of life, but let's talk food. If I told you that you could never eat chocolate again (assuming it's your thang) and you must resort to kale salad for breakfast, lunch, and dinner, you would be thinking about how badly you wanted that chocolate before you even finished the first meal! When your kids are young and they have a play date, they instinctively want the toy their friend wants to play with (even if they don't usually enjoy that toy) because they don't want to feel like it's being taken away from them. The exact same philosophy applies to this process.

If we tell our kids they can no longer eat processed sugar and we remove all of their favorite treats, they will immediately begin finding ways to sneak the candy, cookies, cakes, and muffins back into their diet! However, if you ensure your child feels as though there is an abundance of options for their favorite foods (with inflammatory ingredients or brands swapped out), then they do not feel the instinctual human desire to comfort their feelings of deprivation. For example, if my child likes Fruit Roll-Ups, I might swap them out for BEAR YoYos Real Fruit Roll-Ups, which use no processed sugar. If my child really wants to have graham crackers as a snack after school, I would swap them out with Simple Mills Pecan Cookies, as they have a graham cracker taste, again, without the processed sugar. The trick here is to ensure kids feel like they have an abundance of clean treats so that they never go looking for inflammatory options.

In fact, I tell my kids that because they eat so healthy, they can have extra treats each day. Tosh and Chloe love this because they feel abundance rather than lack. Remember, nutritional health is based *less* on calories in versus calories out and *more* upon the *type* of ingredients going into our mouths each day.

Model First, Then Invite

This last tip is key to successfully get your whole family on the clean-eating train.

So often moms (or caregivers) put others before themselves. I know this all too well. The truth is that we will never be able to help our loved ones in a lasting way unless we first help ourselves in a lasting way as well.

If we want our child to learn how to love and appreciate himself, we must first do the same and model it with ourselves. If we want our son to be a good reader, we must first read with him. If we want our child to be athletic, he is much more likely to be so if we are active with him. If we want our child to be kind to himself, we must first model what that looks like, starting with ourselves.

The same is true with healthy eating. If you want your child to adopt healthy eating habits that last a lifetime, you must first adopt that way of eating for yourself. I have found over and over, both in my life and that of my clients, that when we show up to be the best version of ourselves, we inspire others. It is this inspiration and sense of belonging (with you), that makes family members want to join in on a beautiful journey toward self-growth and healing.

One of my past clients, Trisha, is a mom of four. Her children were in upper elementary and middle school grades. Trisha began working with me to lose weight, improve energy, stabilize hormones, and reduce anxiety. After a couple of months of working together, the contrast she felt in her body from anti-inflammatory eating versus eating her traditional diet was tremendous. She experienced for herself the vitality this way of eating brought to the body, and she wanted to share it with her kids.

At first, Trisha began giving talks about anti-inflammatory eating to her family. She expressed to them how much she truly wanted them to eat healthier and how much better they would feel. None of her kids had any particular health concerns, so there wasn't a strong reason (in their point of view) to change their way of eating. After all, they really enjoyed those cakes, cookies, and slices of pizza! So one day, Trisha made some of the delicious treats from the back of my book, *Peace of Cake: The Secret To An Anti-Inflammatory Diet*. She did not tell her kids they were clean cupcakes, cookies, or pizza until *after* they said, "Hey … these are pretty darn good!" Once her family realized they could still enjoy all of the foods they loved using non-inflammatory ingredients, they were so much more open to enjoying the anti-inflammatory foods that Trisha made at home. Lectures never work, but when people observe you enjoying anti-inflammatory comfort foods, they often want to join the party!

It is when we walk our talk as moms that we model for our children. It is when we walk our talk that we truly understand what it feels like to crave sugar and then how easily we can be satisfied with a clean treat. Or how eating clean protein every few hours melts away all cravings (more to come on that). It is when we walk our talk that we figure out the easiest ways to grab a quick meal on the go, what to pack when traveling on an airplane, how to streamline in the kitchen, and how to manage social settings in a way that is still fun and satisfying. Without first taking care of ourselves, the whole system begins to crumble. Sure, you may be able to add a few food swaps here and there, which is certainly better than doing nothing, but also probably not enough to reverse or significantly improve your child's *chronic* symptoms.

As a mom, it's more than likely that your adrenals are tanked, your metabolism has slowed down, and, because stress has been at an all-time high, comfort food has snuck its way into your life, potentially creating chronic inflammation. That inflammation has gone to those areas most susceptible in your body. Now is the perfect time to reverse all of that.

Imagine what life would be like if you felt vibrant, confident, and energetic while your child experienced freedom from his chronic symptoms. Sound good? I think so! The trick, then, is to adopt this way of eating for a minimum of two weeks – but I really recommend four to nine weeks, enough time for you to experience incredible shifts in your well-being. Enough time for your child to notice how much more patient, grounded, and present you are with him. Enough time for your husband to realize how much more energy you have and maybe even how trim you are looking! The secret ingredient in getting your family on the clean-eating wagon, my friend, is *inspiration*.

The Ripple Effect

This is worth repeating because it is important and vital to changing the lives of people you care about. As I always tell people, anti-inflammatory eating creates a ripple effect. When one person adopts it, very soon others want to know what that individual is doing differently, because that person looks, sounds, and feels so good. As soon as others hear how easy and tasty it is to swap out the top six inflammatory foods, they want to give it a shot too! But it all begins with you, and it requires following through with integrity for at least a couple of weeks so that you can feel the incredible contrast.

The Clean-Eating Kid Tip ————————————————

The four crucial steps to getting your child on the clean-eating train without feeling deprived and without you having to constantly nag them are:

1. Have a discussion to better understand *their why* for changing their diet. How is their chronic condition impacting the way your child wishes to live his/her day-to-day life?
2. Allow your child to become the Renegade Researcher for the family, so he/she can feel in control, and be a part of anti-inflammatory eating, rather than feeling like anti-inflammatory eating is being done *to* them.
3. Provide an abundance of anti-inflammatory treats to ensure no one feels deprived of the foods they enjoy.
4. As a mom or caregiver, adopt anti-inflammatory eating for a minimum of two weeks prior to having your kids join, so that you can model, discuss, and help make connections between what they eat and how they feel. Ultimately, you are being the change you wish to see in your family's life.

Chapter 8

Sugar Withdrawal

What Does Detox Look Like?

By this time, I think you're beginning to understand the negative impact of processed sugar on the body. Interestingly enough, it creates more than just physical challenge. As I mentioned previously, processed sugar has been proven to be as addictive as cocaine. The addiction is real for many reasons, and affects both physical and emotional aspects of the body. In this chapter, you're going to learn how to detox, how to embrace the detox, and what you can do to stop cravings (a common symptom of detoxing) in their tracks.

The goal of our work together is to get as much inflammation *out* of your body as possible. We know there is chronic inflammation lurking in your body. And we know it is in part due to your diet (or you wouldn't be reading this book). We also know that if you keep doing what you've always done, you will continue adding toxins to your body. This means your liver and kidneys will continue to work on overdrive. There will continue to be more toxins than your body can process, and one of two things will happen. Either you will feel more intense symptoms and your health condition will escalate, or your body will create fat pockets to store the toxins as far away from your organs as possible. Neither option is fun, but those are the processes that take place when we cannot get the inflammation out efficiently.

The goal of anti-inflammatory eating is to significantly decrease the flow of inflammation going *into* your body. Then we can use techniques like drinking water, moving your body, Epson salt baths, deep breathing, or meditation and mindfulness to help eliminate any chronic inflammation stuck inside. This is where the detox process truly begins.

Detox occurs when your kidneys, liver, and lymphatic system are pushing out toxins in an effort to eliminate them from your body. The detox process requires your body to process the inflammation (for a second time!) in order to eliminate it once and for all. The effort of pushing out the inflammation can cause an array of symptoms such as headaches, nausea, irritability, tiredness, constipation, diarrhea, brain fog, sleep irregularity, bad breath, achy or flu- or cold-like symptoms, hunger, itchy skin, intense cravings, or bad body odor. Surprisingly enough, this list of symptoms is not complete when it comes to detoxing. If you have a susceptible condition or chronic symptoms, it may rear its ugly head for a couple of days during the detox before it begins to heal. It can sometimes (and very temporarily) feel like you're getting worse before you get better. But I promise you, moving beyond those few days of detox and into the light of regeneration, where the body and mind can begin to work and feel so much better, is a massive milestone. You've entered a new and profound layer of health on the way toward eliminating chronic symptoms.

I once had a client, Sam, who had gout. While the gout did not affect him on a day-to-day basis, it was debilitating when it showed up. As Sam began to eliminate inflammatory foods and swap them out for foods that healed, his gout showed up with a strong vengeance. He was bedridden for two days as his body processed the toxins, but once the major detox was over, the pain went away as well as his gout. He no longer needed medication for gout. While the two days of detox were certainly not the highlight of his life, it was absolutely worth the freedom he experienced as the gout was eliminated from his life.

Often, when people begin to experience detox, they get scared. They may say, "Wait a second. I'm trying to feel better, and I'm actually feeling worse. This isn't working." Or, "I know healing is around the corner, but this feels so crappy I don't want to continue." I want to give you some really good news. The most intense part of detox typically lasts three to five days, and it means you are on the brink of healing and regeneration. Magic begins at the end of your comfort zone.

Detox doesn't last forever, and it's so important to embrace it in order to push through. I love to pivot my thinking during times of detox from, "This is no fun and I hate detoxing," to, "Oh, my word, I've got one raging headache! I'm so tired. And … I'm actually happy about it because I know this means the inflammation is leaving my body." When you are feeling these detox symptoms, you can be assured that the inflammation is getting pushed out of your body. This is awesome, as long you know to think about it in a way that keeps you on the clean-eating train.

The Clean-Eating Kid Tip

NOTE: Because this is a longer chapter, with multiple sections, I'm going to break down each section to provide tips for *The Clean-Eating Kid.*

Detox can look very different for each child, and sometimes the symptoms get worse before they get better. But remember, it's temporary. The lasting positive impact of anti-inflammatory eating on your child will far outweigh a week or two of detoxing. Meltdowns, crying, and tantrums (think of every kid you've seen at the grocery store being denied a candy bar) are extremely common during the detox process. Your child will likely try to convince you that they really *need* a bag of candy, cookie, or whatever treats they are used to having. I promise you that if you hold strong, the crying, whining, and meltdowns will come to an end (although it could take as long as two weeks before their body stops craving processed sugar altogether). This is one of the many reasons why it's important to have a conversation with your child before changing his/her diet.

The more intensely an adult or child detoxes, the more they will crave inflammatory foods. Having extra clean treats on hand to give your child as soon as they crave sugar will help everyone involved. In addition, talk to your kids about what's going on in their body during detox so they understand the cravings won't last forever.

Great job, mama! You are giving your child the gift of knowledge and good health. Beyond your unconditional love, I cannot imagine a more profound and impactful gift.

Stop Cravings in Their Tracks

As mentioned above, in addition to the physical symptoms that one may experience when detoxing, there are the food cravings. A chemical and physiological reaction is taking place in your body during this detox time that makes you crave foods, typically those that aren't good for you. I always know I'm detoxing when, all of a sudden, I want some sort of sugary treat or I want a glass of wine, which is so not how I typically eat. Yet, all of a sudden the craving is real and in my face.

At this point in my life, I'm grateful to be able to notice and observe my cravings, rather than react to them. That takes a lot of practice and often a bit of coaching. So, as you begin this process, I'm going to give you the top three ways that you can stop cravings in their tracks with ease: drink water, eat clean protein, and allow yourself a sweet treat using non-inflammatory sugar.

At the initial onset of cravings, the first thing you want to do is drink a large glass of water. Don't sip on it. Again, throw it back and chug it. Water actually stabilizes your blood sugar levels, lubricates your joints, supports healthy hormone production, and, of course, helps get toxins moving out of the body as quickly as possible. Interestingly enough, I find that when I'm dehydrated, those cravings become stronger. So keep a large bottle of water alongside you and remember to drink, drink, drink it. The bottle of water does you no good if it sits beside you all day, untouched.

Step two is to eat a clean source of protein. After you have drunk a large glass of water (or two), the next step is eat a minimum of 20 grams (for adults) of clean protein. We're going to talk more about what constitutes clean protein in the next chapter. This, too, helps stabilize your blood sugar levels and gives you a sense of grounded-ness. In addition, it supports healthy function of your immune system, fuels your muscles, and boosts your metabolism.

Ultimately, we want to attack the craving by stabilizing your blood sugar levels. When insulin levels are even, so is our blood sugar. This increases our energy and stamina, and allows us to drop the sugar highs and crashes. In addition, stabilizing insulin levels supports the balancing of all of hormones. Many people do not realize this, but removing inflammatory foods and controlling insulin levels is a strategy that has the ability to heal hormone dysfunction. I know this personally, as I was able to get off of Armor Thyroid (a pharmaceutical thyroid medicine) after being on it for six years by following the steps outlined in this book.

The third and last step to stop cravings in their tracks is to give yourself some sort of clean, sweet treat. Remember, this way of eating is not about deprivation. This is not about telling your body you can never have anything that tastes sweet again. This is about giving your body nutrients. It's about fueling your body with sweet-tasting foods that help you regenerate, rather than degenerate, on a cellular level.

So, what does that clean, sweet treat look like? It could be as simple as a pint of berries, a banana, an organic apple, or some sliced up pineapple. It could be one of the delicious, clean, sweet treats that you'll find in Part 2 of this book, treats like Simple Mills cookies, Honey Mama's chocolate bars, or Coconut Bliss ice cream. (You can also find quick and easy recipes in my first book, *Peace of Cake: The Secret to an Anti-Inflammatory Diet*.) When you are detoxing especially, be sure to satisfy your cravings by swapping out inflammatory ingredients for those that do not cause inflammation. It's absolutely my recommendation to make a triple batch of whatever recipe you enjoy eating, or buy more clean grocery swap treats than you think you need. Remember, it's less about *how much* you eat and more about *the type of ingredients* you eat. By having a cache in your kitchen, lunchbox, or office, clean treats are available to you when you have a craving, *right now*. If you have to make the treats, or run to the store, more than likely you will end up reaching for something that makes you fall off the wagon, which has the potential to cause a vicious cycle of negative thoughts and actions that do not support your goal of maximized health.

To recap, we have talked about embracing the detox symptoms, as well as three action steps to stop cravings in their tracks. Number one, chug water. Number two, eat around 20 grams of protein (for an adult). Number three, give yourself some sort of clean treat. These steps are absolutely huge! I have seen people who were lifetime soda drinkers quit drinking soda using these steps. People who were committed sugar-holics, whose diet was 99 percent sugar, eliminated and stopped the cravings completely by following these steps. These steps are transformational, so be sure that you take action, rather than resting in assurance that you know what to do. Knowledge is only one piece of the puzzle in solving your health conditions. *You must take action, as it is in the gap between knowledge and action where so many people fall down.*

The Clean-Eating Kid Tip

Kids crave foods just as often (if not more so) than we do. It is so important for you to practice the steps above so you can offer the same advice to your kiddos. When my kids ask for something sweet, I always respond by saying, "Absolutely! I understand what it feels like to crave sugar. And you can definitely have some as soon as we eat a little bit of quick, clean protein."

You will experience the best results with your kids if eating clean protein sounds quick and easy. Ideally, your child will eat anywhere from 8-15 grams of protein (depending on the age) to steady the craving. This could be an RX bar, 1–2 ounces of grass-fed or free-range meat, one and a half eggs, ¼ cup pumpkin seeds, half a scoop of a high-quality protein powder, *etc.*

And of course, after the protein, be sure to hand over a delicious clean treat!

Five Detox Recovery Tips

Follow my top five tips to help you move through the detox process with more ease and speed!

The first hack to push through detox symptoms more quickly is to take an Epsom salt or Dead Sea salt bath. Get the bath as hot as you possibly can (without burning yourself) and add Epsom salt (following the directions on the container). Sit in that bath as long as you can, allowing yourself to sweat significantly. Sweating is one of the top two methods that helps you push toxins (and fat) out of your body. It is ideal to take a cold shower after the bath, which will continue to help regulate your detox pathways. (And, honestly, it feels really good!)

The second method to support detoxing is through elimination of toxins via urination. This goes back to the importance of drinking *lots* of water, especially if you're feeling less than ideal when detoxing. You have already learned the benefit of drinking one gallon of water each day; however, never is there a more important time to do so than during detox. In fact, if you don't drink enough water while your body is trying to push toxins out, it can actually reabsorb the toxins. *Drinking enough water cannot be emphasized enough.*

A third method for helping to push toxins out of your body more effectively during the detox process is to incorporate gentle movement in your daily routine. I'm not talking long runs, heavy lifting, or high-cardio workouts. The idea is to get your blood flowing, which will help pick up the toxins and inflammation so they can be more easily excreted. Movement such as light stretches, a gentle walk, bouncing on a trampoline, or playing with your child at the park are perfect ways to do this.

The fourth tip is often the most overlooked: *rest*. Rest is one of the lifestyle objectives most important for weight loss and the regeneration of health. It is especially important during detox, as your liver and kidneys are working overtime. Similar to someone who runs a marathon, these organs are exhausted during detox. Expecting them to run a marathon after a night of no sleep is unwise and unhealthy. Rest is a tricky aspect, as sleep can be compromised for a few days at the height of detox. If you are having difficulty experiencing deep sleep, remember that rest counts when your feet are up off the floor and your eyes are closed. Your goal during detox is to carve out as much rest time in your day as possible and begin listening to your body. If it says it's tired, set aside your to-do list and take a cat nap, or put up your feet for as long as you can.

The fifth method for supporting the detox process, and one I highly encourage, is breath work. Deep breathing is another method to remove inflammation from your body. I really enjoy a simple exercise where you breathe in through your nose for three counts and then breathe out for six counts. It is the outward breath that is most detoxifying, although the entire breath calms your nervous system. Find a comfortable place to sit, with your back straight, close your eyes … and breathe. This method tag teams with rest because deep breathing or meditation have been shown to be more deeply restful than sleep itself! So if you are having a difficult time sleeping, try some deep breaths. In fact, you may be surprised at how impactful a short two-minute meditation or breath work session can be. I have witnessed incredible transformations from people who began to incorporate this into their daily routine, myself included.

The Clean-Eating Kid Tip

Detox recovery tips are important for kids as well, and relatively easy to incorporate into their daily routine.

1. When you give your child a bath, be sure to add Epsom salt (as directed on the package). The bath does not need to be as hot for kids as I recommend for adults, but as the kids play with their bath toys, they will have a gentle detox, helping them to feel better quicker. In fact, my kids now request Epsom salt baths – again because I talk to them about how good it is for our bodies. They've learned to listen to their body and request the things that help them.

2. If you know your kiddo is detoxing, encourage them to drink lots of *extra* water, again with fun straws and cups or chugging games!

3. Many kids (unless your child spends more time than not in front of a screen) are quite active. If they are anything like Tosh and Chloe, they're running around morning, day, and night. So it actually becomes more important to encourage them to rest, rather than play hard. You can do this by watching a family movie, taking an extra-long bath, and making sure they get a really good night of sleep. However, if your child typically lives a more dormant lifestyle, then getting them out for a gentle walk, bouncing on the trampoline, or playing on the playground for twenty minutes will help open up the detox pathways to push toxins out. (Too much play can exhaust the body and make it more difficult to detox easily. It's a fine balance.)

4. Meditating moms, you know to encourage your child to breathe deeply. Oxygen, in the form of ozone, is a medical treatment given through a variety of therapies to help the body heal from chronic conditions and support the detoxification process.

5. Any time of the day, we have the amazing opportunity to give ourselves the benefit of extra oxygen by deep breathing – and it's free! If this idea is new to you and your kiddo, trying sitting down and taking seven deep breaths together. I refer to these as balloon breaths with my kids. Have your child sit in your lap (if age appropriate), and place your hand on their stomach. Then tell them to breathe in deeply and to pretend their belly is a balloon that they are trying to blow up. The deeper they breathe, the further your hand will go out. As they let the air out of the balloon, ask them to see how slowly they can let the air out. Follow along, and they will feel your stomach expand and contract if they are sitting on your lap. As you do this, remember that deep breaths where the exhalation is longer than the inhalation have been shown to be deeply detoxifying. It is amazing what a daily practice of seven deep breaths can do to transform each person in your family.

They will sleep better, feel more grounded, be better behaved, and experience an overall deep sense of well-being.

6. Last but not least, I want to discuss a little gene that can make a big impact in the body's ability to eliminate toxins. Over 40 percent of the population has a mutated gene called MTHFR, which blocks the methylation process in the liver and is the foundation of detoxing. While genetic testing to confirm this can cost thousands of dollars, you don't need those tests to take steps to improve your health. There are a few supplements you can take to up-regulate your detox pathways and support the liver's healthy function. I suggest speaking with your doctor about the possibility of taking methylated B complex, glutathione, folate, and any additional supplements that may support the detoxification process. None of this is harmful, and if you have the MTHFR mutation, you will likely notice a change within a couple of weeks.

Chapter 9

Clean Protein Deserves a Food Category of Its Own

We've talked about one of the major action steps to stop cravings in their tracks: drink a glass of water and then eat some clean protein, followed by a sweet clean treat. Clean protein truly deserves a food category of its own, and it's important to understand what I mean by "clean," as protein has the potential to either heal or harm you on a physical level.

Many anti-inflammatory diets recommend not eating meat at all. I understand this recommendation based on the protein that most people in our modern society eat. However, it's important to make a distinction between modern-day meats and the clean protein that we ate for generations. Becoming a vegetarian, vegan, or omnivore is a very personal decision. I'm not here to tell you which category to eat, as each of our bodies function uniquely and thrive from different macronutrient ratios. This chapter is not about whether or not to eat meat, but rather about finding the type of clean protein that best suits you.

Clean beef protein comes from a life lived off of the land, a cow that has only eaten grass or hay, ever. This is important because our food industry now gives cows genetically modified corn and soy as a standard feed. It makes sense. Corn and soy will fatten up cattle much more quickly than having them simply graze off the land. This allows the rancher to sell the cattle more quickly and make more money in an industry that requires tremendous energy, time, and devotion to making minimal money for their effort. The problem is that corn and soy are two of the most genetically modified foods on the planet. It seems that our food industry often comes down to the bottom line. Because genetically modified corn and soy have a higher yield, farmers can sell it to the ranchers for a much cheaper price.

In the following chapters, we will talk in more depth about why genetically modified foods are included among the top six inflammatory foods. What's important to know now is that genetically modified foods are directly linked to leaky gut, which appears in almost all people who have autoimmune conditions. Leaky gut often creates food allergies and ultimately creates a toxic overload systemically, as food is pushed through the intestinal lining and into the rest of the body.

When a cow eats genetically modified food, the toxins and inflammation from the GMO feed enters the body and is typically stored in the animal's fat. When we eat the beef from this cow, we're eating the toxins and inflammation that were stored in the fat and tissues of the cow. This enters our body directly and causes the same havoc in us.

It's important to note that regular, grass-fed beef is not always what it appears. True to the food industry's tricks and misleading ways, it is legal to label beef that has *mostly* eaten grass but then finished on grain as "grass-fed" beef. It's best to look for the label "grass-fed, grass-finished" on beef to ensure you are getting the clean meat you are looking for.

When it comes to poultry, the keywords you want to look for are "free-range organic" chicken or turkey. The term free-range refers to a bird that has been allowed to roam around the fields eating grass and bugs that are chock-full of omega-3 fats. The grass that cows eat and the grubs that poultry eat are full of omega-3 fats, which fight off inflammation in the body. In fact, omega-3 fats are one of the best forms of superfoods available to humans. They help prevent Alzheimer's and dementia. Omega-3 fats help you lose unwanted fat, stabilize hormones, and absorb nutrients through your cell walls.

Fish also requires the art of detection in order to know if it's clean or not. As most of you know, fish, such as salmon, are great sources of omega-3 fats as well. However, that has begun to change in recent times as fish farms often feed fish GMO foods. In addition, fish farms typically do not have adequate space per fish, so they end up swimming around in one another's waste. When purchasing fish, remember to look for *wild*-caught in order to eliminate any inflammatory components within the fish.

Eggs follow the same concept as poultry. Free-range eggs are full of omega-3 and inflammation-fighting fats, while traditional eggs are chock-full of GMO-formed fats that cause inflammation. There has been much debate throughout the years over whether eggs are good or bad for us. The debate has mostly revolved around whether eggs create bad cholesterol in the body. What I find time and time again is that when my clients work on removing inflammation from their bodies (this includes eating an ample supply of omega-3 fats), the bad cholesterol rapidly declines. Again, it is not the egg that is good or bad for you, but the type of egg that determines your outcome. Please note, cage-free is not the same as free-range. Cage-free means it's slightly more humane, and there is less confined space in the pen. Free-range means that the chickens have been wandering around outside, eating grass and grubs.

Why are we talking so much about protein? A lot of people don't get enough protein to fully support or meet their health goals. The minimum amount of protein that best addresses most adults' general needs is approximately 100 grams of protein per day; that's approximately 20 grams of protein every two to three hours. Many adults eat significantly less. The amount of protein a child should eat varies greatly on their age and size, but typically somewhere between 5-20 grams of protein every 3 hours is ideal. Check with your pediatrician for amounts specific to your child's age.

Eating clean protein will help stabilize hormones. It will support the elimination of cravings, which is the most important thing to address if your child is addicted to sugar. It will fill you up and fuel your muscles. Protein supports your immune system and helps you feel more grounded. However, none of this protein does the body good unless it comes from a clean source, so take a little time, speak with your butcher, find your local ranchers, and go to your local farmers' market, where you can source these clean types of protein.

If you are vegetarian, I want to give you a few of the best vegetarian options for getting highly dense protein into your body each day. I recommend eating eggs in the morning as a great source of protein and healthy fat. Each egg is equal to approximately 6 grams of protein. I also love a high-quality protein powder (be sure to read the ingredients to make sure it's free of the top inflammatory foods). Smoothies are an excellent way to use protein powder. Traditionally, one scoop of protein powder is equal to 15-20 grams of protein. Pumpkin and hemp seeds are exceptionally packed with protein. In one quarter cup of these seeds, there are approximately 12 grams of protein. Hemp seeds are *also* chock-full of important omega-3 fats. Sprinkle them on a salad, pour them into a smoothie, or add them to granola, pancakes, and bread. Additionally, legumes can be exceptionally high in protein, depending on the variety.

The Clean-Eating Kid Tip

Throughout this section, you have learned the importance of clean protein. In addition, you've learned how eating clean protein every three hours will stabilize your blood sugar levels, help reboot your metabolism, and cut down cravings. While I do not track how often I feed my kids protein, I always ensure there is a high-quality protein source with each meal and snack that they eat.

The amount of protein ideally consumed by kids is different than adults, and based off of weight. Rather than worrying about or measuring out the amount of protein each child is getting, I encourage you to give them protein before carbs (similar to what you do when a craving hits) to ensure protein is indeed eaten. Remember, carbs are *not* bad for kids. In fact, carbs are absolutely necessary for the appropriate physical and cognitive development of all kids. However, you want to ensure your child is eating a non-inflammatory carb so they can receive nutritionally dense foods that support the body. Kids tend to eat carbs more easily, which is why I encourage giving protein first and then eating some brown rice, baked yam, quinoa, fruit, veggies, *etc.*, second.

Nut-Busting Myths

Contrary to popular beliefs, nuts are not a great protein source. They are a fat source and typically allow you only a couple of grams of protein per serving. The same is true of dairy. While there is protein in it, the primary macronutrient is fat. So if you are eating nuts throughout the day and thinking you are getting your protein in, you will likely want to swap those nuts out for a different source referenced here.

A Day in the Life of Protein – Omnivore

In order to envision what 100 grams of protein per day would look like, check this out. Start your day off with two eggs (approximately 12 grams of protein). Two hours later, make yourself a smoothie with a scoop of protein powder for 20 grams of protein. At lunch time, you might have a salad with approximately 4 ounces of clean meat, maybe some salmon or turkey or thin strips of beef, and a quarter cup of pumpkin seeds. This will give you approximately 40 grams of protein at lunch. As a mid-afternoon snack, you might have a quarter cup of hemp seeds (about 12 grams of protein), and for dinner, you could go for 3-5 ounces of clean meat or fish with some brown rice and roasted veggies (giving you an additional 35 grams of protein). This type of eating throughout the day will give you about 120 grams of protein per day. Of course you can modify this as needed, but this demonstrates the simplicity of allowing yourself enough protein each day.

A Day in the Life of Protein – Vegetarian

In order to envision what 100 grams of protein per day would look like, I have created another sample menu for vegetarians. Start your day off with two eggs (approximately 12 grams of protein). Two hours later, make yourself a smoothie with one-and-a-half scoops of protein powder, for approximately 30 grams of protein. At lunch time, you might have a salad with approximately 2 ounces of goat cheese, a cup of beans, a hard-boiled egg, and add a quarter cup of pumpkin seeds. This will give you approximately 40 grams of protein at lunch. As a mid-afternoon snack, you might have a quarter cup of hemp seeds (about 12 grams of protein), and for dinner, you could go for one serving of organic black bean spaghetti noodles with extra virgin olive oil and roasted veggies (giving you an additional 25 grams of protein). This type of eating throughout the day will give you about 120 grams of protein per day. Use this as a guide to figure out a daily plan that will satisfy your protein needs.

A Day in the Life of Protein – My Clean-Eating Kids

As I mentioned above, I worry less about tracking the amount of protein that my children eat each day, and more about ensuring they are getting some form of clean protein with each meal and snack, as the amount of protein necessary is dependent on age, exercise, and growth spurts. To give you an example, a day in the life of my Clean-Eating Kids looks something like this:

Start the morning with two to three free-range organic eggs. (14 - 21 grams of protein, depending on the child.) As a snack, I give them each a kid's RX bar. (8 grams of protein.) For lunch, I typically give them leftover grass-fed or free-range meat from the night before as a main dish. (1 ounce meat is approximately 7 grams protein.) In addition, I will add Simple Mills crackers, organic fruit, brown rice cakes, carrot sticks, plain goat's milk yogurt flavored with vanilla stevia (around 5 grams protein), and a clean treat. For dinner, we often have sautéed broccoli, grass-fed or free-range meat (again 1 ounce of clean meat is approximately 7 grams of protein), and brown rice or baked yam, sometimes followed by a small serving of Coconut Bliss vanilla ice cream for dessert.

Depending on the day (some mornings we have paleo pancakes instead of eggs, for example, or my anti-inflammatory lasagna instead of meat at dinner), my kids typically eat 30-65 total grams of protein each day, depending on their age and level of exercise. Again, the trick is to ensure they are getting some sort of clean protein with each meal and snack to ensure their blood sugar levels stay stabilized. This will help keep hormone production in balance, even out mood swings, improve cognitive abilities, elevate the metabolism, reduce cravings, and support muscle development through the adolescent years.

Quick Protein Math

- One cup of beans is equal to approximately 7-11 grams of protein.
- Each ounce of meat is equal to approximately 6-8 grams of protein.
- One egg is equal to approximately 6 grams of protein.
- One-quarter cup hemp or pumpkin seeds is equal to approximately 12 grams of protein.
- One scoop of protein powder is equal to approximately 15-20 grams of protein.
- One serving of organic black bean spaghetti pasta is equal to approximately 25 grams of protein.

*There are other sources of protein in which protein may not be the main macronutrient, but there's enough that it certainly adds up over the course of the day. A few examples are steel-cut oats, long grain brown rice, quinoa, spinach, sunflower microgreens, goat cheese, and goat yogurt. (The protein molecule in goat dairy is much smaller and more easily digested versus cow dairy, which is comprised of large protein molecules many adults find hard to handle.)

Chapter 10

Going Deeper: Food Swaps for the Other Top Inflammatory Foods

If you're brave enough to say goodbye, life will reward you with a new hello.
— Paulo Coelho

The Additional Five Inflammatory Foods and How to Swap Them Out

The magic of this process is that by swapping out processed sugar, by default, you eliminate many of the remaining top inflammatory foods: processed wheat, cow dairy, alcohol, inflammatory oils, and genetically modified foods (GMOs). Of course, there are additional inflammatory foods in our world today, foods like sodium, preservatives, and pesticides (which, as an added bonus, are mostly eliminated once you swap out the top six inflammatory foods and purchase organic). Beyond the effects of these top six inflammatory foods, each person responds to unique foods in their own way. The only way to be absolutely certain which individual foods are inflaming you is to hire an anti-inflammatory health coach or to eliminate the top six and, week by week, test the foods that are suspicious. By eliminating the foods that inflame us, we allow the body to be in an environment that supports healing. As an added bonus, removing these top inflammatory foods often causes random food sensitivities and allergies to dissipate.

Approximately every 120 days (give or take some depending on the location in the body), new cells are made through a duplication process in the spleen. This is significant because, if our cells are inflamed, toxic, or lacking nutrients and hydration, they will degenerate throughout the 120 days. Once they get to the replication stage, the spleen will actually duplicate the *degenerative* cell, creating another cell full of inflammation and toxins while lacking nutrition and hydration. Simplistically speaking, this degenerative process is why some people look much older than they are, or why young people end up with chronic illness.

On the flip side, if we begin to eliminate inflammation and toxins from the cells while giving them nutrition and hydration, each cell will become round and plump. Toxins will leave, allowing for red blood cells to absorb vitamins and minerals important to cellular health. As these regenerated cells pass through the spleen, they are also duplicated, this time for the best. The key is to maintain anti-inflammatory eating as well as a healthy lifestyle so you can literally grow young while continuously up-leveling your cellular health.

My goal for you is to get the best bang for your buck when it comes to swapping out foods, so you're eating foods that will make the biggest impact on the inflammation in your body. Replacing processed sugar does just that. If you want to take it a step further, purchase organic foods as much as possible and work at swapping out the remaining top five inflammatory foods outlined below.

Once you have become a master at eliminating processed sugar from your diet, it may be fun to play around with the following foods as you swap them out, and then *listen to how your body responds*. NOTE: I recommend swapping one food out at a time, for at least two weeks, being sure not to eat anything else that you know is inflaming you (like the top six inflammatory foods). Notice if you feel better. Once a food has been out of your diet for one to two weeks, add it back in and *listen to how your body responds.* Do any of those chronic symptoms show up? Do you feel funky in any way? If so, my recommendation is to keep the offending food out of your diet for as long as possible, as my experience and observation is that each of these foods significantly inflames people.

Modern-day Wheat

Wheat is not what it used to be when our grandparents or great-grandparents baked with it. This is largely due to the genetically modified wheat that has overrun our country and other parts of the world. The genetically modified wheat has become a Frankenfood, making many people sick and extra-sensitive to gluten due to the super-injected gluten in each seed.

Beyond the added gluten in highly processed, inflammatory modernized wheat, there is also glyphosate, the active ingredient in Roundup™, found in most GMO seeds. In fact, a recent lawsuit was recently won against Roundup™ linking it to some types of cancer, especially lymphoma. "Bayer-Monsanto has known for decades about the cancer-causing properties of Roundup, and I applaud the jury for holding the company accountable for failing to warn consumers of the known danger," stated Ken Cook, president of the Environmental Working Group, after the trial.

The story of a Wheaties-type cereal will shed some light on how wheat has been turned from food into a food-like product. Once upon time, hunters and gatherers learned how to grow crops, which helped them settle in one location to create their own civilizations. During this time, people would plough the land with animal and manpower. There were no tractors driving over the earth back then or fertilizers being added to the ground.

People would plant wheat seeds that had been plucked from their neighbor's fields. There was no Roundup™ embedded within the seed to ensure its ability to grow and beat the chances of insect destruction. There were also no hybridized seeds injected with extra gluten. The likelihood of this seed surviving was purely up to nature. If the wheat plant made it to maturity, someone would harvest the plant. The wheat was then brought to someone who specialized in grinding the wheat using a bowl and tool made out of stone. This was extra tricky because unlike modern wheat, which gets pumped full of gluten to make the wheat fluffy, ancient wheat was small and coarse. The wheat would get mashed up between two stone objects until it turned into a wheat meal of sorts. (Kind of like almond meal.) This is what our ancient relatives used to bake bread with. The bread was not light and fluffy. In fact, it was thick and dense – much like what you find when you purchase Ezekiel non-GMO sprouted wheat bread.

Today, the Wheaties (or insert any modernized wheat product) that so many of us use and know well is made from wheat that doesn't deserve to be classified in the same category as ancient wheat. Once the Roundup™-laden seed is planted into the already chemical-soaked soil, it sprouts and matures (consistently). Due to the GMO process, this wheat is supercharged with extra gluten, ensuring our breads, cereals, and pastries have an extra-fluffy consistency. In turn, the extra gluten in each wheat plant over-exposes us to gluten, causing a host of inflammatory conditions. Once harvested, the chemically and genetically altered wheat is taken to a facility where it is heated up, chopped up, and spit out as a plant our body no longer recognizes as food.

Modern-day wheat is found in a host of random, food-like products. It can be found hidden in everything from soups and vodka to lipstick and envelope adhesive. Modern-day wheat, along with cane sugar, soy, and corn, is among the top genetically modified foods on this planet. We're going to talk more about genetically modified foods in the next section, but it's important to note there are multiple reasons why wheat causes inflammation for people.

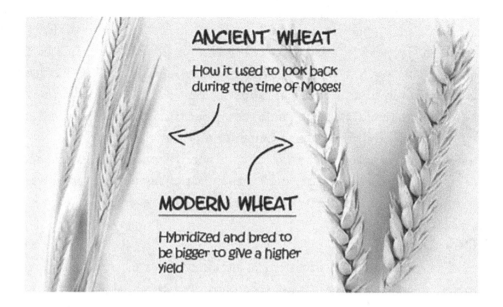

ANCIENT WHEAT

How it used to look back during the time of Moses!

MODERN WHEAT

Hybridized and bred to be bigger to give a higher yield

Wheat Food Swaps

Everyone's unique make-up determines what their body can tolerate. However, I have found that small amounts of an ancient sprouted wheat in a bread that uses no processed sugars, cow dairy, or other inflammatory oils works well for most people. Of course, the key is listening to your body to see if symptoms arise after eating the ancient sprouted wheat. NOTE: If you have an autoimmune condition, it is probably best to stay away from wheat altogether until your body heals.

One of the food swaps I love to give my kids to replace modern-day wheat bread is the previously mentioned Ezekiel Bread. Ezekiel Bread is a more dense bread (much less gluten), and is made from sprouted grains, which means it is less processed. You can find it in the freezer section of most grocery stores. In addition to all of these benefits, Ezekiel Bread is one of the few grocery store bread options without processed sugar. It tastes fabulous toasted with extra virgin coconut oil spread over the top. For a fluffier bread, try making my Fluffy Sandwich Bread, a recipe you can find in my first book, *Peace of Cake: The Secret to an Anti-Inflammatory Diet*. This recipe is grain-free, mixed in a blender, and then baked. It doesn't get much easier to make bread than that.

Some additional wheat swaps are coconut paleo wraps for sandwich rolls and sprouted, non-GMO corn tortillas for tortilla swaps. In Part 2 of this book, you will find recipes for pancakes, muffins, cakes, cookies, pizza, and more using coconut and almond flour as wheat flour substitutes. Last, I love to use Tinkyada organic brown rice pasta as a traditional pasta replacement. While there are a number of different gluten-free pastas out there, I find Tinkyada pasta to most consistently replicate the experience of traditional pasta in texture and taste. In fact, many of my clients swap it out at home, and their families never know the difference!

Cow Dairy

Lactose is a naturally occurring sugar found in cow dairy. When found in its natural form, lactose is not the culprit that causes large amounts of inflammation in the body. However, the processed sugars such as corn syrup, cane sugar (even if it's organic), and other inflammatory sugars often found in flavored dairy are the exact sugars you want to stay away from. Beyond the sugar, cow dairy is inflammatory for other reasons. To begin with, the protein molecule in cow dairy is quite large. It's so large that our body doesn't easily digest it.

Beginning at birth until around the age of three, our body creates extra digestive enzymes that help break down larger protein molecules. This bodily function is created from an evolutionary process. In primitive caveman times, people would breastfeed their children until around the ages of three or four. To adapt to a larger intake of milk, infants and toddlers are able to digest cow milk because their bodies have the necessary digestive enzymes. Slowly, as they mature, children become less capable of breaking down the larger protein molecules.

Beyond the size of its protein molecules, cow's milk also creates inflammation because of the feed the cows are given – usually, genetically modified corn and soy. The inflammatory properties of GMO corn and soy enter the cow's body, including the milk. When we ingest that milk, either alone or as yogurt, ice cream, or cheese, it, in turn, inflames us. You may wonder if grass-fed cow dairy would be a better option. My answer is, yes, however you still have to deal with the large protein molecules and yet another issue, below, that causes inflammation in the body from cow dairy.

Cow dairy's issue number three that causes inflammation are the hormones and antibiotics commonly used by dairy farmers. In order to ensure cows provide enough milk for long enough periods of time, cows are often given growth hormones and antibiotics. Similar to beef, these hormones and antibiotics are passed on to the consumers eating the dairy products.

Cow Dairy Food Swaps

There are a number of cow dairy swaps that work really well. As a milk alternative, I prefer organic canned coconut milk, goat milk, or homemade nut or seed milk. The reason I recommend either canned coconut milk or homemade nut/seed milk is because many of the milk alternatives found in boxed cartons are full of inflammatory oils, preservatives, and often sugar.

When swapping out yogurt, I love either goat or sheep yogurt. Both of these yogurts need to be purchased in their plain form, without sugar. My trick to add a bit of pizazz is to mix approximately three droppers of vanilla crème, mixed berry, lemon, or orange-flavored liquid stevia into one serving of plain yogurt. To add even more depth of flavor, find a food-grade essential oil and add two to three drops of lemon or orange essential oil with the complementary stevia flavor. Mix in some organic frozen berries, and you have one delicious treat, packed with a substantial amount of clean protein.

Cheese is often a food people really miss when eliminating cow dairy. Luckily, in recent years an array of goat and sheep cheeses has become available. Goat cheese is no longer defined as just that stinky, soft cheese crumbled onto salads. You can now find cheddar, mozzarella, and even jack-flavored goat cheese. I specifically use the brands Alta Dena and Mt. Sterling goat cheeses to melt on quesadillas, grilled cheese sandwiches, and lasagna. Manchego sheep cheese is another favorite that can be shredded and melted for a slightly richer flavor. NOTE: Many of the nut and rice cheese substitutes use canola oil or other common inflammatory oils.

The last cow dairy swap that is near and dear to many people's hearts is ice cream! While I have only found one company that uses non-inflammatory sugars, they have many flavors and are absolutely delicious! Coconut Bliss ice cream seems to stand in integrity with their ingredients. They are also easy to find in local grocery stores. So go ahead and have a guilt-free bowl of ice cream on me.

A quick note about goat and sheep dairy, and why the body responds better to it. The smaller the animal, the smaller the protein molecule found in the dairy. This is important because we have digestive enzymes that can more easily break that protein down. In addition, because it's goat and sheep, it likely doesn't have the same antibiotics and hormones as that of cows (although that may be changing as the demand for goat and sheep dairy increases). Lastly, goats and sheep are traditionally set out to graze rather than fed GMO feed, though again note that this trend could potentially change with the increase in demand for goat and sheep dairy.

Alcohol

Alcohol itself is highly inflammatory, and while this book is titled *The Clean-Eating Kid*, I know that by now you are understanding the need to first adopt anti-inflammatory eating as a caregiver before you ask your child to do the same. So, in the spirit of helping parents and kids alike, we will address the top inflammatory drinks most common to people of all ages: alcohol, juice, and soda.

To begin with, let's talk about wine, beer, and cocktails. Alcohol turns into a sugar in our body and is tied with processed sugar for the number one inflammatory food. Unfortunately, it can be one of the trickiest foods to swap out, as it is tied so closely with social settings and one's desire to unwind after a long day. There is a slew of conflicting information with regard to alcohol and whether or not it is good for you. Remember, my focus is primarily on eliminating inflammation from the body. While there are excellent health benefits that can be reaped from the antioxidants found in the grapes used to make wine, sadly the alcohol wipes out much of the good that comes from the antioxidants.

Beyond the problem of alcohol causing massive amounts of inflammation, I have a few fun facts about wine that just may make you think twice before picking up your next glass. Fifty-one percent of all US wine is actually manufactured by three giant wine conglomerates. There are 76 chemical additives approved in the US by the FDA for use in making wine, including copper, ammonia, and many more.[11]

US wines are often made with genetically modified commercial yeast. Ninety-nine percent of US vineyards are irrigated and fed synthetic fertilizers. Monsanto's Roundup™ is the most common herbicide used in US vineyards today. Top-selling approved additives used by the US wine industry include "mega purple," which is a coloring agent, and residual sugars, fructose, and glucose, are commonly left present in wine to appeal to the US consumer's sweet palate. Sugar in wine can be as high as 300 grams per liter! And beyond that, glyphosate (the herbicide linked to cancer) was recently found in ten out of ten wines from California including organic and biodynamic wines![12]

I realize wine is not the only source of alcohol, yet I find it to be the most commonly debated topic in the world of nutrition in terms of whether or not alcohol can be good for you. Rather than debate semantics, I challenge you to a science experiment. Eliminate alcohol completely for two weeks to see how *your* body responds. (It takes approximately two weeks for the inflammation from alcohol and processed sugar to pass fully through your body.) At two weeks, determine how you're feeling. Are your chronic symptoms reducing, or gone? If so, it's no coincidence.

Often this experiment is easier than people think. I once worked with a woman named Katie who was 23 years old and lived in a ski town that knew how to party. She was single and loved to go out on the town with her friends, yet she had a deep desire to also take care of her body by following an anti-inflammatory diet. Katie decided to participate in a little two-week science experiment to see how good she felt when not consuming alcohol. After two weeks, she was convinced that she wanted to continue living this way. She felt much more grounded and in control of her life.

In order to have fun and maintain this lifestyle while still socializing with friends, Katie discovered a trick that made it easy to be social and enjoy herself without drinking alcohol. The trick was to have some sort of fun cocktail glass filled up with sparkling water (maybe even a tiny splash of cranberry juice) and a twist of lime. The key was to have it in an actual cocktail glass of some sort. What she discovered was that drinking was much less about the alcohol itself, and much more about feeling a sense of belonging with a group of people. When you have a fun mock-tail in your hand, not another soul needs to know it is non-alcoholic. Even if you are not drinking for a social occasion, simply having something special like a unique and fun mock-tail to sip on at the end of the day is often just as satisfying as an alcoholic cocktail itself.

Katie was able to go out on the town and attend all her many social engagements with her friends without ever feeling like the odd duckling. She set an example of *living*.

Alcohol Swaps

I believe there are three key components to swapping alcohol out of your diet. Number one, make a drink that you do not often have. Something that, like a glass of wine, you may traditionally only consume one time at night. An example of this is purchasing coconut water and then add a few mint sprigs and a couple of raspberries to your glass. It could also be sparkling water with a splash of juice (not from concentrate) and a twist of lime. You could even muddle up some berries and mint, add the combination to sparkling water, and mix in a few drops of vanilla crème stevia. You get the idea. It's about having fun and being creative with a drink that you do not drink often. The second key component is putting your drink in an actual cocktail glass of some sort. For example, I like to pour organic coconut water with mint sprigs and raspberries into my great-grandma's crystal wine glass. It feels so special and celebratory! The last key component is to always have a plan or mock-tail with you when you know you will be in social settings. Similar to clean eating, when we don't have a plan or swap available to us, it is significantly more challenging to stay on the wagon.

Juice, Gatorade, Soda, and Sugary Drinks

I'm adding a special category for juice, soda, and sugary-kid drinks as they are just as inflammatory as alcohol itself and often consumed even more frequently.

While juice concentrates, sugar in Gatorade-like drinks, and soda are wildly different beverages from each other, they are all made from the number one inflammatory food, processed sugar. And if you think the work-around is diet soda or sugar-free options, think again. In fact, studies published in *The American Journal of Clinical Nutrition* show that artificial sugar substitutes can potentially increase your chance of cancer, increase weight gain, and cause metabolic syndrome, type 2 diabetes, and cardiovascular disease.

According to a study conducted by the Centers for Disease Control, roughly two thirds of all children consume at least one sugary beverage on any given day, and roughly 30 percent consume two or more a day.[13] Remember the idea of "everything in moderation"? Is one sugary beverage per day considered moderation? And if so, what does that mean when we see processed sugar for what it is, a toxic drug? That's a lot of chemicals we are allowing our children (or ourselves) to consume each day.

Sugary Drink Swaps

First and foremost, it's so important to remember that juice concentrate is a processed sugar and is representative of the number one inflammatory food you can put into your body (remember, there are over 50 names for processed sugar). Even though I share this with my clients all of the time, it still surprises even me! Pear juice concentrate just *sounds* so benign. Needless to say, it is not. So when choosing the perfect juice for your family, I only recommend considering a freshly squeezed, not-from-concentrate option.

Many health food groceries will squeeze fresh orange juice in the store directly for your purchase. It is also fun to buy a juicer and make your own apple, watermelon, or orange juice with your kids. Juicing at home is a great way to get the whole family involved, and is the perfect opportunity to make clean, anti-inflammatory popsicles for the summer months. In fact, I have an amazing watermelon popsicle recipe in my first international bestselling book, *Peace of Cake: The Secret to an Anti-Inflammatory Diet*. Be sure to grab a copy so you can make these for yourself – I can't keep the watermelon popsicles around long enough during the summer months!

If you are looking for a stepping-stone to wean yourself from soda, my recommendation is Zevia soda. While it still has some preservatives that I'm not over the moon about, it is a wonderful swap for traditional soda, which is full of inflammatory ingredients and chemicals. Once you are ready to move on to the next soda swap, try plain sparkling mineral water with 3-5 drops of liquid stevia flavors such as vanilla crème, berry, blood orange, or lemon. It's great-tasting, simple, and has no added preservatives. Win-win for all!

A great way to swap for a Gatorade-like electrolyte drink is to purchase a liquid flavorless electrolyte (with no sweeteners or preservatives). You can find these on Amazon or at your local health-oriented grocery store. If you want to add a bit of taste, try one of the many different liquid stevia flavors such as grape, orange, lemon, *etc*. Also, coconut water is a terrific electrolyte source, and if you want a drink with some natural sugar as a pick-me-up after athletic training, this is the perfect choice. There are many wonderful options, but Harmless Harvest cold-pressed, non-GMO, organic coconut water is my favorite. (Plus, it's naturally pink, which makes the perfect juice swap for your little princess in the house.)

Refined Oils

Refined oils are similar to processed sugar in the sense that it is easier to focus on what you can eat, rather than what does not work. Generally speaking, vegetable oils cause inflammation, as do many seed oils that are heated. Last, trans-fats are not only inflammatory, but also illegal in most countries because of their extreme toxicity. Contrary to common thinking, fats do not make you fat and sick. Just like clean protein has the ability to heal the body, so do anti-inflammatory oils such as organic, extra virgin, cold-pressed olive, coconut, and avocado oils.

Avocado and coconut oils can be heated at higher temperatures, so they are ideal for cooking. The higher the polyphenol content (an antioxidant) found in olive oils, the stronger the anti-inflammatory properties they hold. When you eat the right oils, you support your body's ability to absorb nutrients at a cellular level, boost healthy hormone production, increase your metabolism, and even help prevent Alzheimer's and dementia.

Genetically Modified Foods (GMOs)

When we eat food, our body is designed to scan the DNA in that food to identify whether or not the food is indeed something the body welcomes, or a potential invader. Genetically modified foods have DNA that has been altered from the original state we were intended to eat. When we consume these genetically modified, food-like products, our body perceives a threat. This puts the immune system in overdrive, ultimately compromising its effectiveness. In addition, GMO foods have been directly linked to Leaky Gut, a condition linked to most autoimmune conditions and digestive disorders.

The most common GMO foods are corn, soy, cane sugar, wheat, and canola oil. Unless labeled *certified non-GMO*, these products are almost always GMO, so be sure to look for that label.

The Clean-Eating Kid Tip

The most important thing you can do for the health and well-being of your child is to completely eliminate processed sugar and swap it out for the alternatives mentioned in this book. Once you have a handle on this, it will be much easier to swap out each of the additional top inflammatory foods, because many of them will have already fallen by the wayside.

If you are generally looking to be proactive and ensure your child's good health, then simply swapping out inflammatory sugar may be all you need to give your child an amazing start in life. However, if your kiddo has a chronic condition, closing the door to each of these top inflammatory foods can be the difference between seeing a *slight* improvement versus watching a health condition begin to reverse. If you plan on swapping all of the top inflammatory foods out, start with one thing – processed sugar. Become a Renegade Researcher, and once your family has perfected that (or close to it), move on to one more food, such as dairy. Take each food one step at a time, rather than eliminating them all at once, so that no one feels overwhelmed.

Chapter 11

A Two-Week Science Experiment

The Challenge

Congratulations, you have made it through the meat of this book (no pun intended), and are ready to put knowledge into action. This is the most important step, because all too often we find ourselves bursting with knowledge, yet lacking time, motivation, and follow-through for implementation. It is this gap between knowledge and action where I find so many fall down. Take a moment now to make a commitment to yourself and your family. Commit to taking action, right in this moment. In the world of "diets," tomorrow never comes, and there's always a reason to start later. But is there a good reason to allow your health, and that of your family, to degenerate for even one more day? Results only show up with consistent action. Give yourself two consistent weeks to determine just how much better your body can feel by adding water and removing processed sugar from your diet.

Once the two weeks are up, begin those conversations with your children, and share with them how much better you feel and how much better of a mom you have become. Congratulations! Point out that you are more patient, energetic, and fun to be around. Ask if your kids would be willing to support you by joining this way of eating, and help them find *their why*. Share that they get to be Renegade Researchers for the family and help pick out fun new foods that taste good and help our bodies grow big and strong (replace big and strong with *their why*).

Remember, the first step is all about you. By first taking care of yourself for two weeks, you will be more patient and kind, feel less stressed, have improved energy, enjoy better sleep, and have less pain and bloating (to mention a few benefits). Beyond that, you will learn to walk your talk, which is *everything* in helping your child make connections between what he/she eats and how he/she feels. Ultimately, this is the most precious gift. When your child is old enough to eat what he wants, he will be able to make informed choices by listening to his body, rather than grabbing whatever is available. You taking care of yourself is where it all begins.

I know that, as moms, putting ourselves first can feel counterintuitive. Remember when Tosh was so sick as a baby? I was so scared. I was a first-time mom, my baby had been sick for over a year – chronically sick, deathly sick – and we were back home. For the first time, my body was processing all that had taken place, and I started to become sick. All of the stress from the previous year was finally showing up in my body, and it looked like an auto-immune condition. Had I not taken the challenge to first take care of myself, I never would have made it to the step of changing my son's diet and significantly helping to heal him.

I watched my mom, who had had chronic Lyme disease for twenty years, heal by changing her diet and working with an anti-inflammatory health coach. My mom modeled this way of eating for me, and it is because she stepped up to the challenge that I was inspired to model it for my children. What an incredible legacy to leave behind – passing on health and regeneration for three generations. Don't you want that for your family too?

In this two-week challenge, you will experience what it's like to go from craving sugar to stopping cravings in their tracks, simply by eating clean protein every few hours and drinking more water. I want you to experience the freedom of eating clean treats as a way to feel satisfied and stop the deprivation. My wish for you is to experience how fun it is to find new and exciting foods in the grocery store or recipes. Clean eating really can be fun and easy. I am so excited for you to experience first-hand how chugging a bunch of water in the morning actually makes you thirstier, and how, by doing this one step at a time, you begin to push inflammation out of your body, gain energy, eliminate joint pain, and likely even lose a few pounds on the scale.

I have watched entire families commit to this two-week process and shift everyone's diet, from adults to middle schoolers to young children, of their own free will. I have watched senior boys in high school reduce anxiety and depression, improve ADD, and improve academic achievements and athletic accomplishments. I have witnessed a three-year-old who had been chronically constipated suddenly experience regular bowel movements. I have seen a young boy struggling with an eating disorder find a new relationship with food, gain healthy weight, and improve his athletic performance. I've watched a middle school-aged boy come out of depression, overcome lack of interest in school, and move toward regular engagement and excitement about his education. I've seen insulin levels from diabetes significantly drop, even halve. I've seen moms drop ten pounds, gain energy, and begin to reverse chronic conditions. I have watched entire families begin to regenerate the cells in their body while initializing the reversal of autoimmune conditions. A commitment to two weeks – just 14 days – can be incredibly powerful.

Two weeks. Give it your all. Stay in integrity and watch the magic unfold. Two weeks is a blink of an eye through the lens of a lifespan, yet it has the potential to become the most impactful and significant two weeks of your life.

As caregivers, it is our job to step up, to model, and to become a source of inspiration for our children. It is when they see that we are more patient and calm, that we're more grounded, that we feel so much better and have all of this energy and time available at the end of the day to play with them on the playground and read them books, and when they see you enjoying the tastes of these foods, that they will reach the point of buy-in and want to join you on this journey. This process is all about coming together as a family, rather than pushing something on someone else. I have learned the hard way that when we try to push this way of eating on someone else, it often backfires in our face. So be the change you wish to see in the world. Try it for two weeks. Get really, really excited about it. Share it with your family and invite them in. I can't wait to find out what magic awaits you all!

The Clean-Eating Kid Tip

After you have conducted this two-week science experiment on yourself, invite your kids in, and ask them to also sign on for two weeks. This gives an "end" date that will make it feel less like a big, scary, life-changing shift. It's more of a fun family challenge. Once the two weeks are over, you can talk as a family about how much better you feel and what it would be like to continue with this way of eating.

Chapter 12

Navigating Social Events and Holidays

Rather Than Deny, Educate

Before we delve into my tips for navigating specific social events, there is one overarching message I would like to share, which is to always educate and make connections between food and the body, rather than to deny your child. I know I've mentioned this before, but the number one thing that makes us (and our kids) fall off the clean-eating train is feeling deprived. Most of the time, when my kids ask for something, we have a conversation about how it impacts their bodies. I try to make direct connections and give examples that they can relate to. For example, Tosh will sometimes ask for a slice of pizza at our Whole Grocer. My response will often be:

"Do you remember the last time you ate pizza? It tasted really good at first, and then you got super tired, your tummy hurt, and then it became extra difficult to make good choices. In fact, remember how you had a consequence for not listening? As good as it might taste, I really want to help you have a great day! What else can we get that tastes good and supports your body?"

This response is very different than a hard no. Instead, I am helping Tosh make direct connections by reminding him how inflammatory foods impact him, and then inviting him into the conversation to find an alternative. If he responds by saying he wants to buy paleo cookies instead, I am going to let him (even if he's eating a treat before a meal in this case), because I want to demonstrate the importance of clean food over inflammatory food. Also, he will feel like he *is* getting a treat by eating cookies first, all while allowing his chronic condition to continue to improve.

I apply this same concept when attending social events. My kids and I will have a planned discussion before going to a birthday party, attending a Christmas festival, or even participating in a holiday like Halloween. We make a conscious decision about what they will eat, and based on that, we will bring food swaps to these events accordingly. However, if it's super important for my child to have a slice of birthday cake, we will once again discuss how it makes him feel. If my child is still insistent upon it, then I will ask if he's willing to drink extra water, eat lots of healthy protein (we know the cravings will hit hard after he eats that cake), and stay super clean for two whole weeks. I remind him that it takes two weeks to get the inflammation and toxins from the cake out of his body and that I'm cool with him eating the cake, if he's cool with not feeling so well afterwards. I also ask Tosh to then promise me that he will eat super well for 14 days so we can get back to a place of regeneration in the body. I find this to be a great compromise, and an opportunity for kids to connect the symptoms they feel with the foods they eat.

Which leads me to my last important piece of advice. When my child is following through with a two-week challenge of totally eliminating inflammatory sugar, then I ask that he/she stick to that. Whether you are just starting anti-inflammatory eating for the first time, or your family fell off the wagon and is ready to hop back on, it takes two weeks to push the toxins and inflammation out of the body from these top inflammatory foods. Without following through with integrity for those two weeks, you (and your child) will not feel the contrast in your body and mind to really notice how much better you feel.

So often, people walk around feeling much worse than they realize. Allow yourself and your children the gift of two weeks so that you can experience the contrast of vitality and regeneration. This way, if your child does choose to have a slice of birthday cake, he/she can truly feel how it makes them feel. Beyond all of the tips and tactics I teach in this book, helping your child learn how to listen to the symptoms in his body and correlate it with diet is the most important lesson. It is this skill that inspires us to continue *living* a healthy lifestyle for life.

General Theory for All Social Events and Celebrations

Generally speaking, my rule of thumb at all social events and celebrations is to supply food swaps for myself (and my kids). For a birthday party, we will bring our own cupcakes. For Christmas celebrations, we make our own cookies. For after-school sports, I grab a bar or snack that I know my kids love (or pack extra in their lunch). In addition, I tell the instructor/coach that my child has a food allergy and has his own snacks packed in his lunchbox. (It's always good to let all adults in on the little secret.) Teachers love to give out rewards at school, and unfortunately, these are often candy. At the start of each year, I bring in Simple Mills cookies, Smart Sweets (gummy bears made with stevia), or Heavenly Organics Peppermint Patties (made with honey). The teacher keeps a stash of clean treats so if she is rewarding the class with candy, my kids have a healthy (yet delicious) swap.

A fun tip for adults: if you are going to a dinner party or barbecue, my trick is to always bring a substantial dish that you know you can eat. For example, you could bring your own grass-fed hotdogs (see part two of the book), a pasta salad made with Tinkyada brown rice pasta, your favorite clean dessert, fruit salad, or some potato chips made with avocado oil and non-GMO ingredients.

The Clean-Eating Kid Tip

When it comes to celebrations, events, and rewards, the feeling most kids experience when trying to follow an anti-inflammatory diet is isolation: being left out. It's very important to ask for your kids' input – what their favorite treats are that they would like you to leave with their teacher, for example. In addition, always make sure they have more than enough food after practice so they are not left feeling hungry with nothing to eat. Beyond those suggestions, *have fun* finding new healthy food swaps or trying out some new recipes together in the kitchen!

Chapter 13

Obstacles: Watch Out for Falling Rocks!

A s you adopt anti-inflammatory eating, there will be obstacles that fall into your family's path. You guys will likely take a trip, go out to eat, attend a birthday party, celebrate a holiday, or simply feel tired and unprepared for dinner one night. Life happens. There will be times your grandma or mother-in-law makes you cookies and tells you how much it means to her if you eat them. You will have to face moments when your friends think you're crazy to eat this way and teachers judge you for how strict you are. It is your conscious decision about how to handle these situations that will often determine success or failure.

Starting anti-inflammatory eating (especially if you follow my process written in this book) is truthfully quite easy. The difficulty is much less in adopting anti-inflammatory eating, but more so in maintaining the way of eating that allows you to feel vibrant, mentally and physically, for extended periods of time.

Typically, when we fall off the wagon, a whole slew of thoughts begin to surround us. It is in fact not the cookie we ate or the wine we drank that determines success or failure, but rather the thoughts we think when these things occur, as they directly predict the next action step that will either bring us back to the clean-eating train or, alternatively, take us on a downward spiral of binging on ice cream, cookies, and treats.

Here's how it works. The most common thing that triggers a craving is some sort of event. The event doesn't have to be a big, prominent event. It could be as simple as your husband looking at you funny, or your child back-talking. That event will automatically create a thought in your mind. Typically the thought shows up so fast that we don't even know it was formed, but might look something like: *If I had more energy, lost a few pounds, or were more fun, my husband wouldn't look at me that way.*

The thought immediately creates an emotion, which in this example would align with defeat, depression, frustration, *etc*. Now, here's the direct correlation between our thoughts and the foods we eat. The moment we feel a negative emotion (also known as stress), we begin to have cravings. The cravings don't show up with slow and moderate intensity. They show up *now*, and three seconds of time seems far too long to wait to satisfy that craving with a sweet treat. The problem is, once we eat, we quickly feel guilty for having done so. We realize that our action likely compounded the problem of not having enough energy, being unable to lose weight, or feeling less than ideal. As soon as those thoughts show up, more negative emotions and, therefore, more cravings appear. Pretty soon, not only is our mental and emotional stability out of alignment, but we also start to have chemical reactions in our body due to the processed sugar, which jump-starts physiological cravings. (This is the time to implement the three steps to stop cravings in their tracks.)

With your family, and alone as a parent and caregiver, it is very rewarding to take note of and bask in your achievements. Emphasize the mental, emotional, and physical health you are creating for yourself (and your family) when you swap out these top inflammatory foods. *Feel* how much more connected you have become as a family. Notice the grounded-ness, patience, and overall family fun that may not have been as predominant in the past. You are doing such incredible work!

However, when you do have a negative thought – and you will – practice lengthening the amount of time between the thought and any food-related reaction. See if you can push past the need for a sugary comfort food or drink, or at least give yourself a clean swap.

The best way I have learned to increase the space between thought and unhealthy treat is to take seven deep breaths the second I am aware of a negative feeling or craving. You can try it yourself: breathe all the way down into your belly, and then breathe out. On your outward breath, try to breathe for double the time you breathed in. For example, breathe in for three seconds and out for six seconds. Modify the time to a pace that feels good for you. This type of breath work is detoxifying, and seven breaths is just enough time to create the space you need between the thought and the reaction to allow yourself a more optimal option. Once we can see that we want the cookie/cake/soda/wine, *etc.* because we are looking for comfort, we have a greater chance of reaching for our healthy food swap, which will create a positive cycle of feeling empowered. This, in turn, gives us a greater chance of repeating the new healthy habit in the near future.

Here's how the cycle goes that creates a negative experience based on the thought you *choose* to have.

An EVENT (The kids won't stop throwing a fit ... lots of screaming and yelling.)

... becomes ...

A THOUGHT ("This is driving me crazy. I just need a break and to have my own peace and quiet.")

... which becomes ...

An EMOTION ("I feel stuck, hopeless ... I can't run away from my own kids!")

... which turns into ...

A REACTION ("I'm stuck in this mess, so I might as well have a glass of wine or chocolate cake to soothe the pain.")

... and then creates ...

A NEW THOUGHT ("Darn it! I *was* doing so well with my diet. Now I've screwed it up. Might as well indulge some more!")

... And the cycle continues.

Let's try a positive twist on this to see if we can get ourselves out of a pickle and feeling empowered.

An EVENT (My kids won't stop throwing a fit ... lots of screaming and yelling.)

... becomes ...

A THOUGHT ("This yelling is loud, and almost becoming comical! What can I do to help both my child and I get through this situation with more ease and grace?")

... which becomes ...

An EMOTION ("I feel empowered, and my brain is being trained to find a solution rather than focus on the problem.")

... which turns into ...

A REACTION ("I am going to take seven deep breaths outside on the porch, then walk in and tell my child that I know he's really upset, and if he wants some snuggles to feel better, I am here for him. If I still feel an emotion of frustration, I may walk into the kitchen and pour myself a wine glass of *kombucha* and eat a clean cookie to give myself the satisfaction that I feel I need in that moment.")

... and then creates ...

A NEW THOUGHT ("I feel proud of myself! My child feels loved, and I know I can make it through other stressful situations by choosing thoughts that best support me.")

... And the cycle continues.

Feeling Better

One of the reasons I love anti-inflammatory eating is because you feel better really quickly. Within two weeks of becoming a Renegade Researcher and truly eliminating processed sugar while increasing your water intake, your life could be completely transformed. And the better you feel, the more you want to celebrate. Celebrating each small (and big) step is a crucial component of this process. However, it is important to choose celebrations that reflect healthy living rather than celebrating how good you feel with a pint of Ben and Jerry's. Ironically, the better you feel, the less motivation you sometimes have to continue eating an anti-inflammatory diet.

A past client, Kim, recently shared her story with me. She had been diagnosed with cancer a number of years ago and quickly changed her diet, which she religiously maintained for a solid year. After incredible healing, Kim began to slowly eat foods that inflamed her, because she no longer had the motivation to eat quite as well. She was in remission and she felt *so much better.* Bit by bit, one piece of pizza at dinner turned into weekly meals. Three bites of chips at a party turned into daily road snacks. Her once-perfect score of drinking a gallon of water each day turned into a few glasses. Alcohol showed up for weekly cocktail hour, and trips to the ice cream store were too good to pass up. All of the little bites here and there became "gateway drugs" that slowly led back to old ways of eating. Along with the old food habits came past symptoms. Kim's energy declined significantly. Her stomach seemed constantly bloated. She tried to go back to an anti-inflammatory diet, but it felt so hard. She was caught up in a story, the story that eating clean was hard. The truth is that there is nothing easier than grabbing some fruit from the store, a few organic nuts, and some clean protein to munch on. It's less expensive and time-consuming than going out. The truth is that clean eating is as easy as it gets, from a logistical point of view.

Food truly has the ability to heal our body. The confusion often lies between connecting our symptoms with the foods we eat. When people go to the Mayo Clinic or other major healing centers, they are often told they have an inflammation-based condition, but are not always given a name for it. They feel hopeless and are desperate to get their lives back on track. They have tried different diets to support their health, only to find it improves their symptoms minimally. Sometimes these people have been able to make large and impactful shifts in their diet, but maintaining that method of eating is unrealistic. They fall off the wagon, which triggers more inflammation in the body and exacerbates the symptoms. This adds to the feeling of hopelessness. The correlation between healing and diet becomes incredibly confusing, and they don't know where to turn.

Luckily, if you know there is inflammation in your body, then following my anti-inflammatory protocol will, by default, support the elimination of the inflammation, hence freeing up the symptoms that suck up all of the resources available to you. The tricky aspect to following an anti-inflammatory diet is that there are no governing bodies or set regulations determining what an anti-inflammatory diet really is. If you Google "anti-inflammatory diet," you will find people sharing anti-inflammatory recipes using organic cane sugar and whole wheat flour! Some people define eating an anti-inflammatory diet as simply adding many of the anti-inflammatory spices (such as Ceylon cinnamon, turmeric, black pepper, cayenne, ginger, garlic, *etc.*) into their diet. These spices absolutely have anti-inflammatory components and are fabulous to add to your cooking. However, if you have not eliminated the top inflammatory foods and swapped them out with ingredients that allow the body to heal, you will not eliminate the root of the problem.

The Clean-Eating Kid Tip

As I've discussed throughout this book, learning how to really listen to your body, understanding why symptoms are showing up based on the foods (or lack of water) that you've consumed, and adjusting accordingly is the golden ticket toward health and vibrancy. First you must walk your talk so you can be the best role model for your child. The more you learn about yourself and how food is connected to your health, the more health benefits you will be able to share with your child. When we give up on ourselves, we ultimately give up on our family. We are a pillar of strength for our families. Without a strong pillar, we cannot fully support those we love.

Grocery Store Food Swaps

In Part 2 of this book, I'll show you many of the anti-inflammatory foods my family buys that are perfect swaps for favorite kid foods. For example, try swapping out traditional chips (like these below) for NON-GMO potato chips made with avocado oil. Both are chips, and both are tasty, yet one will allow your cells to regenerate while the other will wreak havoc in your body. The key to maintain anti-inflammatory eating is finding food swaps that taste delicious while simultaneously ditching the inflammation.

It's amazing how long the book writing and publishing process takes. By the time this book was written and published, more delicious and healthy food companies sprouted up that I want you to know about! So be sure to visit **www.cleanfoodswaps.com** for a more robust list of anti-inflammatory grocery store food swaps.

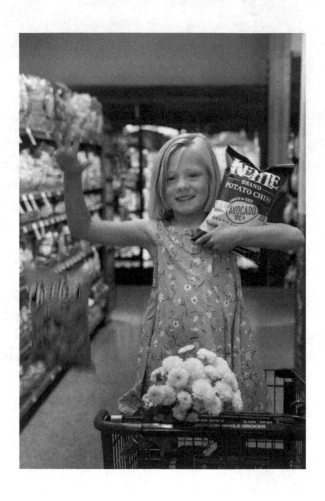

Take a Peek Inside My Grocery Cart with These Grocery Store Food Swaps

Note: Visit **www.cleanfoodswaps.com** for the newest anti-inflammatory grocery store food swap options that have emerged since the publication of this book. Bonus! You'll get to download a free guide to help you make grocery shopping easy and quick, while choosing foods that help your family feel great!

In the pages that follow, you will discover a sample of my family's favorite food swaps that you can find at the grocery store, online at Thrive Market (which I find to consistently be most cost-effective) on Amazon, or in many of your favorite health food stores. These grocery store swaps are free of the top six inflammatory foods, allowing you more time in your day to enjoy the things most important to you.

SUPER IMPORTANT: While I have chosen to highlight food companies that make healthy eating a priority, *it is essential that you continuously check the ingredients labels on the foods you buy.* Small companies often get bought out by large companies, or recipes slightly change, and both have the potential to add inflammatory ingredients to the foods you buy. These swaps are intended to get you looking in the right direction with companies that care, so continue being a Renegade Researcher as you navigate your way through the grocery aisles. In fact, even within food companies, the difference from one flavor to the next can determine whether or not inflammatory ingredients are used. Keep your eyes peeled and *have fun* exploring the foods that these forward-thinking companies are supplying us with.

A note to the reader: Know that not all brands are created equal. A food like cauliflower pizza crust sounds healthy and amazing, but there are a variety of manufacturers out there. Always read the ingredients – are you seeing a theme here? For example, Cali'flour Foods Cauliflower Pizza has four simple ingredients for their plant-based pizza crust, while a different brand such as Caulipower, has 14 ingredients (many of which are inflammatory). Both are cauliflower pizza, but they are not nutritionally the same. So as you go throughout these swaps, you will see specific brands and flavors I recommend, you will find inspiration to dig deeper at your grocery store, and hopefully you will discover even more options for you and your family!

Produce Section

A quick note on the produce section. Ideally, you want to stick to organic fruits and vegetables, especially if they fall under the dirty dozen list of the most pesticide-ridden produce. Beyond that, anything here goes. The more fruits and veggies you eat, the more nutrients your body has access to, including cancer-fighting nutrients such as antioxidants.

A recent study conducted by the United States Department of Agriculture found 230 different pesticides on thousands of different products. In addition, the Environmental Working Group analyzed USDA pesticide residue data and found that almost 70 percent of non-organic produce sampled tested positive for pesticide contamination. And more than 98 percent of samples of strawberries, spinach, peaches, nectarines, cherries, and apples tested positive for residue of at least one pesticide.[14]

You may be asking yourself the same question I did when I read about pesticide residue. How harmful can a little residue be? That question was answered by the Environmental Working Organization, a non-profit, non-partisan organization.

"Several long-term studies of American children initiated in the 1990s found that children's exposures to organophosphates – not only in farm communities but also in cities – were high enough to cause subtle but lasting damages to their brains and nervous systems. Children with higher concentrations of organophosphate and pyrethroid pesticides in their bodies are more likely to be diagnosed with ADHD.

"Between 2014 and 2017, EPA scientists re-evaluated the evidence suggesting organophosphate pesticides affect children's brains and behavior. The EPA concluded that ongoing use of one pesticide, chlorpyrifos, was not safe and proposed to ban the chemical. However, shortly after taking office, EPA Administrator Scott Pruitt cancelled the scheduled chlorpyrifos ban and announced that the agency would not finish its safety assessment for chlorpyrifos until 2022.[15]

"A group of recent studies suggest an association between consumption of fruits and vegetables with higher pesticide residues and fertility issues. The Harvard EARTH study found that men and women who reported more frequent consumption of high-residue produce had fertility problems. At the same time, the amount of lower pesticide residue fruits and vegetables in their diets was not associated with negative effects. The researchers have also detected similar fertility impacts in younger men."

I pause to share this information with you because the produce section is the one area where my "secret" to an anti-inflammatory diet does not apply. Whole fruit is amazing for you, yet being aware of pesticides and the neurotoxins that they release into the body directly impacting inflammation and chronic symptoms is extremely important. Below, you will find a list of the dirty dozen foods, of which I highly recommend purchasing the organic version. In addition, you will find a list called The Clean 15, which are fruits and vegetables least likely to contain pesticide residue.

Dirty Dozen List

- Strawberries
- Spinach

- Nectarines
- Apples
- Grapes
- Peaches
- Cherries
- Pears
- Tomatoes
- Celery
- Potatoes
- Sweet Bell Peppers

Clean 15

- Avocados
- Sweet Corn (NOTE: Be cautious of corn for its GMO properties)
- Pineapples
- Cabbage
- Onions
- Frozen Sweet Peas
- Papayas
- Asparagus
- Mangos
- Eggplants
- Honeydews
- Kiwis
- Cantaloupes
- Cauliflower
- Broccoli

Pasta, Rice, and Soup Aisle

Tinkyada Brown Rice Pasta is our family's favorite pasta swap! It is made with brown rice (be sure to choose the organic version), and, unlike many other gluten-free pastas, it has a beautiful al dente texture. In addition, Tinkyada offers a variety of different pastas such as lasagna (find an anti-inflammatory lasagna recipe in my first book, *Peace of Cake*), spaghetti, penne, spirals, linguini, and shells. Delicious for homemade mac-n-cheese, too!

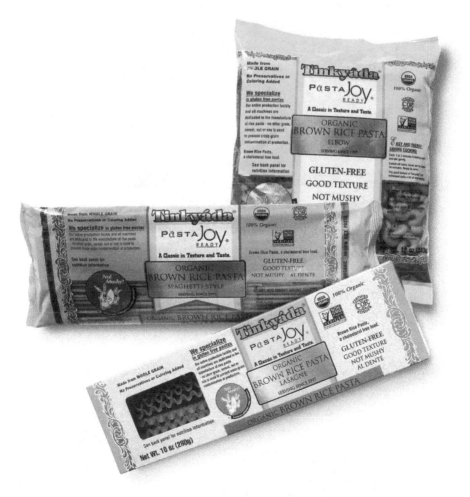

Ingredients: Stone-ground organic brown rice, rice bran, and water

Capello's is a fun paleo egg noodle swap! Find these in the freezer section of your grocery store, and enjoy another flavor and texture of clean pasta that your kids can't resist! Best part – these delicious pastas come in many styles and textures, like fettuccini, lasagna sheets, and even a fun gnocchi!

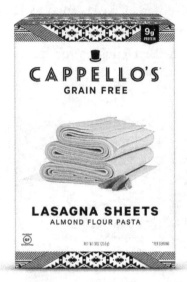 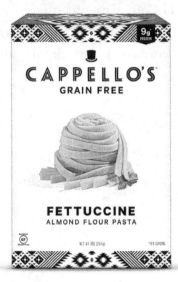

Ingredients: Almond flour, cage-free eggs, tapioca flour, xanthan gum, sea salt

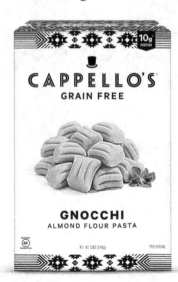

Ingredients: Organic potato, almond flour, cage-free eggs, tapioca flour, sea salt

Amy's Organic Lentil Soup is my son's favorite soup swap! Full of protein and free of processed sugar (which is difficult to find with canned soup), it is a nutrient-dense and simple meal on a chilly day.

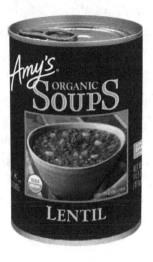

Ingredients: Filtered water, organic lentils, organic celery, organic carrots, organic onions, organic potatoes, organic extra virgin olive oil, sea salt, bay leaves

Lundberg Long Grain Organic Brown Rice is the perfect swap for all other rice. Long grain means it's less processed, and organic is extremely important for brown rice, as arsenic can be readily found in non-organic rice. Cook this with a little virgin coconut oil and sea salt for a delicious flavor.

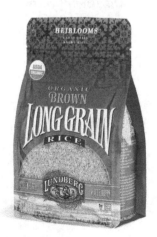

Ingredients: Organic brown rice

Frozen Pizza and Crusts

Cali'Flour Foods pizza crusts are the best way to sneak some added vegetables into your family's diet! These pizza crusts are unlike any cauliflower pizza I have seen – both in taste and quality. Unique to this brand, their pizza crusts have whole foods without the fillers. Beyond pizza crust, Cali'Flour pizzas can be used to make crackers, lasagna sheets, and more! There are a number of different flavors, but to keep cow dairy out of your diet, I recommend the vegan or plant-based option. You won't regret it!

NOTE: Cali'Flour Foods pizza crusts are showing up in more and more grocery stores, but you can always purchase and have them shipped directly to your home by going to https://www.califlourfoods.com.

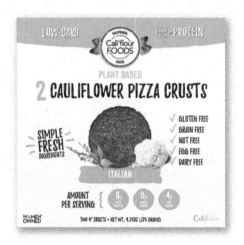

Ingredients: Fresh cauliflower, almond flour, flax meal, olive oil, tapioca starch, garlic powder, dried basil, Himalayan pink salt, nutritional yeast

Bean, Salsa, and Tortilla Aisle

Green Mountain Gringo Salsa prides themselves on making a clean salsa, which I personally am grateful for! This salsa is not only free of processed sugar (often found in salsa), but it's also free of preservatives!

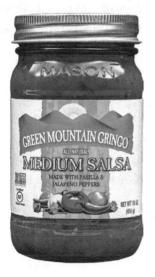

Ingredients: Ripe tomatoes, fresh onions, tomatillos, apple cider vinegar, fresh jalapeño peppers, fresh pasilla peppers, cilantro, parsley, fresh garlic, sea salt, cumin

Siete Tortillas are my new favorite swap for flour tortillas. The owner of Siete is on her own healing journey, which drives the inspiration and quality of Siete foods. These tortillas have a very similar texture and color to flour tortillas (sometimes important to kids) and come in three amazing flavors: almond flour, cassava and coconut flour, and cassava and chia.

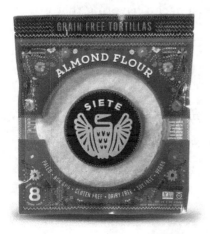

Ingredients: Almond flour, tapioca flour, water, sea salt, xanthan gum. Ingredients vary depending on the flavor.

Crackers, Chips, "Crunchies," and Jerky Aisle

Simple Mills Crackers are my kids' favorite crackers swaps. The sea salt flavor reminds me of traditional saltine crackers. You can also choose from more mature flavors such as rosemary, sundried tomato & basil, and farmhouse cheddar (which is cow dairy, so I tend to leave that flavor on the shelf, but may be a good transitional swap for goldfish-type crackers).

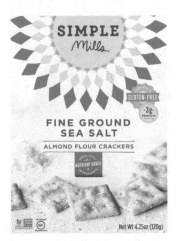

Ingredients: Nut and seed flour blend (almonds, sunflower seeds, flax seeds), tapioca, cassava, organic sunflower oil, sea salt, organic onion, organic garlic, rosemary extract (for freshness)

Siete Grain Free Tortilla Chips are hands-down the best swap for traditional tortilla chips. These taste amazing, yet are made with non-inflammatory ingredients and cooked in avocado oil (which can be heated to high temperatures before becoming inflammatory). For those of you who love Dorito-style chips, Siete makes a nacho flavoring that is totally clean and super tasty!

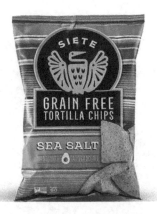

Ingredients: Cassava flour, avocado oil, coconut flour, ground chia seeds, sea salt. Ingredients vary depending on the flavor.

Lesser Evil Organic Popcorn is my favorite popcorn swap. I often send this treat to my kids' classrooms for popcorn parties. It's also a favorite finger snack for picnics and birthday celebrations. I love this brand because they use non-GMO corn, which is very important, as well as high-quality avocado or coconut oil.

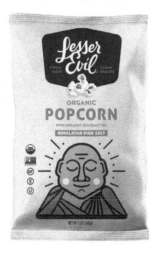

Ingredients: Organic non-GMO popcorn, organic coconut oil, Himalayan salt. Ingredients vary depending on the flavor.

Quinn Microwave Popcorn is a great swap if your child is trying to make hot popcorn for a movie night with friends. Also made from non-GMO corn, this popcorn is popped without any oils. I prefer the Sea Salt flavor as an anti-inflammatory swap.

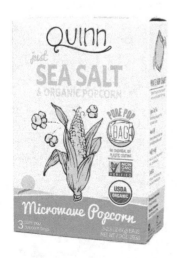

Ingredients: Organic popcorn kernels, sea salt

Lundberg thin, thick, or round rice cakes are the perfect swap for a healthy snack on the go and are chock-full of carbs that will support your child's growth. I especially love that Lundberg's rice cakes are organic and non-GMO. There are many flavors, including brown rice with sea salt, red rice and quinoa, and more! Be sure to double-check that you are buying a flavor without processed sugar.

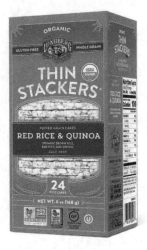

Ingredients: *Organic brown rice, organic red rice, organic quinoa. Ingredients vary depending on the flavor.*

Nature's All Natierra freeze-fried organic strawberries and pineapples are a fun swap for any sweet and crunchy snack you may be looking to replace. Packed with antioxidants, these are a real treat to eat on their own or add to cereal. Best of all, they are light and easy to tote around and are bursting with delicious flavor!

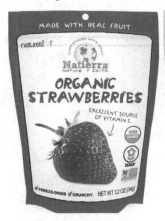 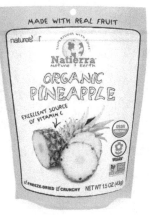

Ingredients: *Organic strawberries or pineapple*

Mary's Gone Crackers have been one of my long-standing favorite cracker swaps. These organic, gluten-free, whole grain vegan crackers come in a variety of flavors, with the Super Seed being my favorite, as it is a great source of clean protein.

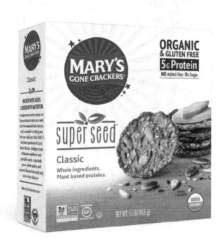

Ingredients: Organic whole grain blend (organic whole grain brown rice, organic whole grain quinoa, and organic whole grain millet), organic pumpkin seeds, organic sunflower seeds, organic brown flax seeds, organic brown sesame seeds, organic poppy seeds, filtered water, sea salt, organic seaweed, organic black pepper, organic herbs. Ingredients vary depending on the flavor.

Go Raw sprouted flax snacks are another great chip or cracker swap bursting with zest and a nice crunch. These come in a variety of flavors such as zesty pizza, spicy fiesta, sunflower, plain, chewy apricot, banana bread, pumpkin seed, raisin crunch, and sweet spirulina. With all of those options, each member of your family can find their favorite snack.

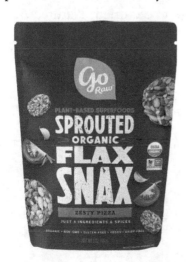

Ingredients: Sprouted organic flax seeds, sprouted organic sunflower seeds, sprouted organic sesame seeds, organic tomato, organic tomato powder, Celtic sea salt. Ingredients vary depending on the flavor.

Epic has become one of my favorite "beef" jerky swaps, after meeting the owner at a conference a few years ago. This company is passionate about providing clean meat that comes from large-scale grassland restoration efforts. While there are many flavors, the bison meat flavor is free of processed sugar, which is commonly found in jerky-type meat products. Great for car trips, backpacking, or river floats, these are the perfect way to get your protein in.

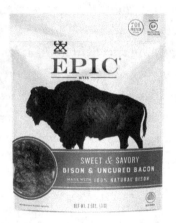

Ingredients: Natural bison, uncured bacon (pork, water, sea salt, vinegar, celery powder), golden raisins, chia seeds

Nature's All Natierra organic, freeze-dried beets recently became my most treasured chip or cracker swap. These are crunchy and light with a mild hint of sweetness. Even better, beets are known to cleanse the blood. For any root vegetable, it's especially important to eat organic, and while there are a number of brands that advertise freeze-dried, Nature's All is free of inflammatory oils.

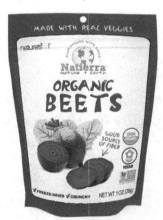

Ingredients: Organic beets

Cookies, Brownies, and Treats Aisle

Go Raw Ginger Snaps are perfect if you love ginger snaps as much as I do! These cookie/cracker treats are mildly sweet with a bit of zest! Loaded with healthy carbs and fats, you can rest assured your family is supporting every cell in their bodies each time they pop one of these into their mouths!

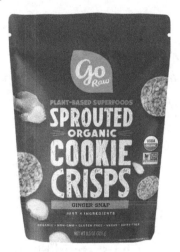

Ingredients: Organic coconut (un-sulfured), sprouted organic sesame seeds, organic dates, organic ginger

Simple Mills Pecan Cookies are a great swap for graham crackers! Boasting a similar taste and texture to graham crackers, they are perfect for a semi-sweet snack. And to make this swap even sweeter, you can find Simple Mills cinnamon and chocolate chip flavors to boot! (The chocolate chips in the chocolate chip cookie do use processed sugar, so be sure to read the ingredients.)

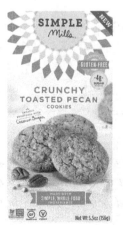

Ingredients: Nut flour blend (almonds, coconut, tiger nuts), tapioca, organic coconut oil, organic coconut sugar, arrowroot, vanilla extract, cinnamon, baking soda, sea salt, konjac root, rosemary extract (for freshness), cream of tartar. Ingredients vary depending on the flavor.

Jack's Paleo Kitchen Lemon Zing Cookies are another delicious treat (because all kids need options for amazing sweets without the inflammatory ingredients). Jack's Paleo Kitchen cookies come in a number of delicious flavors without inflammatory ingredients: lemon zest, cinnamon raisin, ginger molasses, nut-free trail mix, snickerdoodle, and sunflower seed butter!

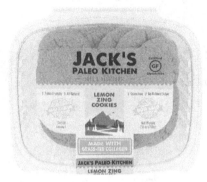

Ingredients: proprietary flour blend (organic coconut flour, arrowroot powder, sweet potato flour), organic palm shortening, honey, maple syrup, water, apple cider vinegar, lemon oil, grass-fed collagen, baking soda, salt

Honey Mama's chocolate bars make me feel like I'm eating a treat at the spa! These incredible chocolate bars boast anti-inflammatory ingredients, and unlike most of the dark chocolate found in grocery stores, these are 100 percent free of processed sugar. To top it off, Honey Mama's comes in an array of different flavors: Peruvian raw, coco-no-nut, Dutch, Mayan spice, Oregon peppermint, lavender red rose, nibs and coffee, ginger cardamom, and so many more! Find these online or in the refrigerator section of your grocery store.

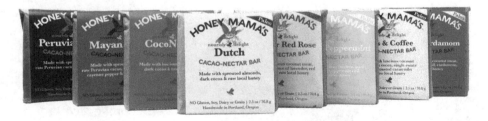

Ingredients for Oregon Peppermint flavor: Single origin alkalized cocoa, Oregon heirloom peppermint oil, raw local honey, coconut meat, unrefined coconut oil, and Himalayan pink salt. Ingredients vary depending on the flavor.

Hu chocolate recently became one of my favorite chocolates when my kids and I found one of their chocolate bars in the airport during a long layover. We were thrilled to find a clean treat at an airport (traditionally not known for health food)! Within the last year, Hu has rocked out an entire line-up of chocolate like quinoa crisp (my favorite), Orange Dream, Salty Dark Chocolate, Crunchy Mint, and so many more.

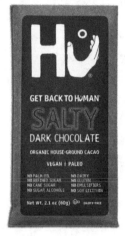

Ingredients: Organic cacao, unrefined organic coconut sugar, organic fair-trade cocoa butter, sea salt. Ingredients vary depending on the flavor.

Hu Gems are the *perfect* swap for chocolate chips. And we can't have clean-eating kids without some delicious chocolate chips! Brand new to the market, these won't disappoint. Whether you add them to your favorite cookies, or munch on them by the handful, I hope you thoroughly enjoy them!

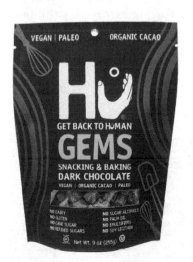

Ingredients: organic cacao, unrefined coconut sugar, organic fair-trade cocoa butter

Hail Merry Tarts are ridiculously delicious and the perfect swap for any celebratory treat. You can even put a candle in the tart and eat it as a birthday cake! These can be found in the refrigerator section of your grocery store, and come in a number of different sizes as well as amazing flavors such as chocolate almond butter, coconut vanilla crème, dark chocolate, Meyer lemon, chocolate mint, and Persian lime.

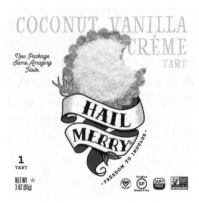

Ingredients: Organic shredded coconut, organic extra virgin coconut oil, organic maple syrup, organic coconut water, natural raw almond flour, organic palm sugar, raw cashews, organic Madagascar bourbon vanilla, sea salt

Oils and Baking Aisle

Nutiva offers an excellent organic, cold-pressed, virgin coconut oil. One of the benefits of coconut oil is that it can be heated to high temperatures without causing an inflammatory response. It's the perfect swap for butter, canola oil, or vegetable oil.

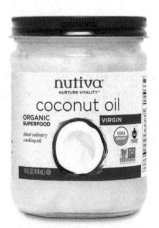

Ingredients: Organic, unrefined, cold-pressed, extra-virgin coconut oil

Primal Kitchen avocado oil can also be heated to a higher temperature, which makes it another excellent swap for butter, canola, or vegetable oil. With a smooth and subtle flavor, avocado oil is a great substitute for refined oils in just about any recipe out there.

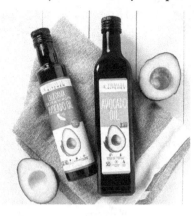

Ingredients: 100 percent pure avocado oil

Coconut Secret Raw Coconut Vinegar is a delicious and light salad dressing swap. A low-glycemic vinegar made from the sap of coconut blossoms, it is similar in flavor to apple cider vinegar.

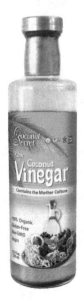

Ingredients: Organic coconut sap naturally aged for eight months to one year

Simple Mills Pancake and Waffle Mix is an everyday staple at our home. This amazing mix is the perfect swap for your traditional pancake batter. Simple and quick to make, your kids will love Sunday morning pancakes made by Simple Mills.

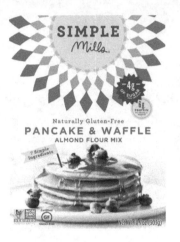

Ingredients: Almond flour, arrowroot, organic coconut sugar, organic coconut flour, cream of tartar, baking soda, sea salt

Birch Benders Pancake and Waffle Mix is another great swap for your traditional pancake or waffle batter. In particular, these pancakes are extra fluffy, which my husband loves, and is quick to make (which I love).

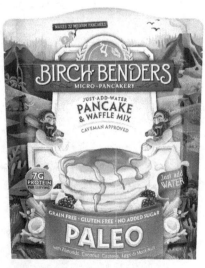

Ingredients: Cassava flour, organic coconut flour, almond flour, eggs, leavening (monocalcium phosphate, sodium bicarbonate), salt, monk fruit (a non-inflammatory natural sweetener), spice

Simple Mills Artisan Bread is the quick, easy, and non-inflammatory way to swap out traditional dinner rolls with homemade bread baked in no time. Super tasty with lots of healthy ingredients. Your family will thank you for this one!

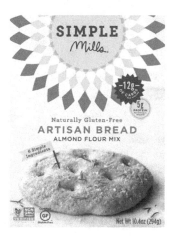

Ingredients: Almond flour, arrowroot, flax meal, tapioca, sea salt, baking soda

Namaste Pizza Crust is the perfect swap for both pizza crust and homemade bread sticks. Add pizza toppings, or add extra virgin olive oil, crushed garlic, and goat mozzarella for a real treat!

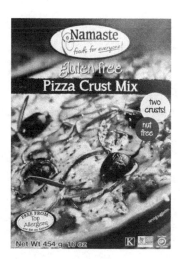

Ingredients: Brown rice flour, tapioca flour, arrowroot flour, xanthan gum, granulated garlic, cream of tartar, salt, baking soda, Italian seasoning (garlic, onion, oregano, rosemary, thyme, basil, sage, marjoram), citric acid

Simple Mills Pizza Dough! I know how much kids love pizza, so I'm adding as many options as possible for you to enjoy!

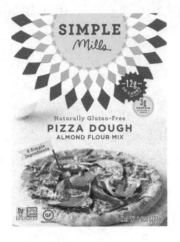

Ingredients: Almond flour, arrowroot, flax meal, cauliflower, baking soda, organic oregano, cream of tartar, organic garlic

Namaste Muffin Mix is a fabulous base to add your own spin to muffins or scones. It's delicious, with add-ins such as bananas, walnuts, coconut sugar with cinnamon, pumpkin and spices, or blueberries and honey. Have fun with all the combinations!

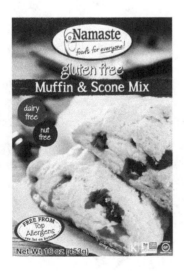

Ingredients: Sweet brown rice flour, brown rice flour, tapioca starch, arrowroot powder, rice milk powder, cream of tartar, baking soda, salt, xanthan gum, ground vanilla bean

Bob's Red Mill has an abundance of alternative baking flours such as pecan flour, almond flour, coconut flour, and more. While it takes a little playing around to figure out the right texture depending on the flour you are using, these are all incredible non-inflammatory baking options.

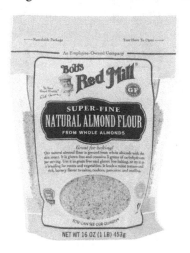

Ingredients: Blanched almonds. Ingredients vary depending on the type of flour.

Otto's Cassava Flour is an amazing grain-free alternative to traditional flour that can be swapped for the same 1:1 ratio, meaning one cup of wheat flour can be traded out for one cup of cassava flour. In addition, cassava flour gives baked items that fluffier and slightly stretchy texture that you experience in traditional breads, doughnuts, and muffins.

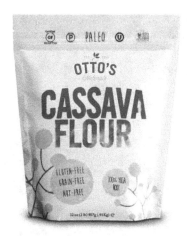

Ingredients: 100 percent cassava (yuca root)

Simple Mills premade muffin mix is the perfect swap for your traditional muffin. Only requiring a few additional ingredients, this is a delicious item to stock in your pantry for last-minute baking options. You can find these in pumpkin muffin and banana bread flavor.

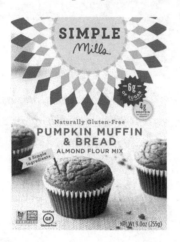

Ingredients: Almond flour, organic coconut sugar, pumpkin, arrowroot, organic coconut flour, organic spices (cinnamon, nutmeg, cloves), baking soda, sea salt. Ingredients vary depending on the flavor.

Simple Mills makes these delicious *chocolate* muffin and cupcake mixes. Their low-key sweetness is better suited for the muffin lovers out there, so if you're looking to turn this into a cake, I recommend adding a bit more non-inflammatory sugar.

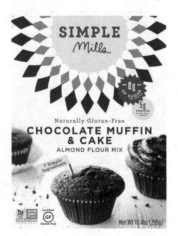

Ingredients: Almonds, organic coconut sugar, arrowroot powder, cocoa, organic coconut flour, baking soda, sea salt

Simple Mills Vanilla Cake and Cupcake mix makes birthday parties super easy. Just as with the chocolate cupcakes, I typically add a bit more clean sugar along with a little vanilla extract to make them extra-delicious!

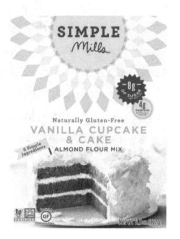

Ingredients: Almond flour, organic coconut sugar, arrowroot powder, organic coconut flour, baking soda, sea salt

Bars, Cereal, and Granola Aisle

Rewind Bars are my favorite bar out there, and one of the greatest secrets in the grab-n-go bar department! These bars are relatively new to the market, and made by a company with incredible integrity when it comes to using high-quality ingredients. I especially enjoy that **Rewind Bars** are not only free of inflammatory ingredients but also chock-full of super foods. Now available in a host of delicious flavors such as Coconut Chocolate Chip, Mocha Latte, Cinnamon Coffee Cake, Almond Butter and Jelly, Mint Chocolate Chip, and, of course, their Original flavor, these bars can only be found online at **http://www.rewindtoday.com**, but I promise – it's worth the trek to your computer.

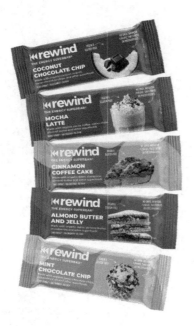

Ingredients: Spinach, kale, almond butter, cashew butter, strawberries, blueberries, cherries, pea protein, spirulina, green tea, chlorella, dates, quinoa, coconut, cocoa. Ingredients vary depending on the flavor.

One Degree Sprouted Brown Rice Crisps are the perfect swap for Rice Krispy-type cereals. Add a dollop of pure maple syrup with unsweetened almond milk for a delicious breakfast. Your kids will love these!

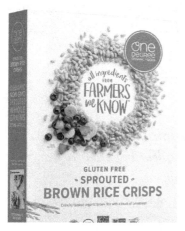

Ingredients: Organic sprouted whole grain brown rice, organic coconut sugar, unrefined salt, tocopherols (vitamin E)

Purely Elizabeth is not only the perfect granola swap for cereal, but also an amazing snack for any lunchbox. My son loves to eat the clusters of granola as a sweet treat! Purely Elizabeth comes in a number of different flavors, however the original is definitely my favorite (but you'll have to try them all and tell me what you think)!

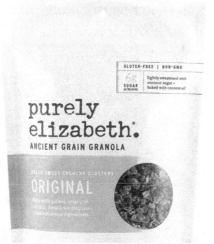

Ingredients: Organic certified gluten-free oats, organic coconut palm sugar, organic raw virgin coconut oil, organic puffed amaranth, organic quinoa flakes, organic sunflower seeds, organic chia seeds, organic cinnamon, sea salt. Ingredients vary depending on the flavor.

Love Grown Original Power O's are an amazing Cheerio's swap! One of only a few breakfast cereals free of inflammatory ingredients, these are made with beans, which also pack loads of protein into each bowl. Add raw honey or pure maple syrup for a little sweetener, and be sure to purchase only the *original* flavor if you want to stay clear of processed sugars.

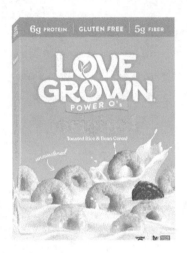

Ingredients: Bean blend (navy beans, lentils, garbanzo beans), brown rice, salt, vitamin E (to maintain freshness)

Bread Aisle

Julian Bakery Paleo Bread is an excellent swap for pre-made, grain-free bread. You can find these in three different flavors: Coconut, Almond Flour, and Seed Medley. Likely found in the freezer section of your local grocery store (or online). Perfect for grab-n-go sandwiches.

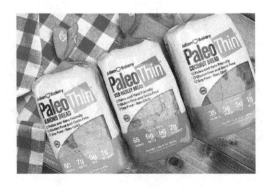

Ingredients: Purified water, almond flour, organic coconut flour, egg whites, psyllium seed powder, organic lemon juice, potassium bicarbonate, sea salt

Dave's Killer Bread is the perfect transition for kiddos who still crave the fluffy texture of traditional wheat bread, but need a healthy option. While Dave's Killer Bread does have gluten in it, if your body can support organic whole wheat, this is the only non-GMO, traditional bread free of any other inflammatory ingredients, including processed sugar and refined oils. Added bonus – there are about five grams of protein in each slice! **Note:** The POWERSEED flavor is the only option I've found to be free of processed sugar.

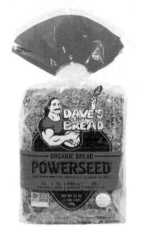

Ingredients: Organic whole wheat (organic whole wheat flour, organic cracked whole wheat), water, powerseed mix (organic whole flax seeds, organic ground whole flax seeds, organic rolled oats, organic sunflower seeds, organic pumpkin seeds, organic un-hulled brown sesame seeds, organic un-hulled black sesame seeds), organic wheat gluten, organic fruit juices (organic apple, organic pear, organic peach), organic oat fiber, sea salt, organic cultured whole wheat, yeast, organic vinegar

NUCO Coconut Wraps are an incredible bread and tortilla swap if you're looking to ditch all bread and tortillas and head straight for a one-ingredient wrap! These are pliable, subtly sweet, and ultra-delicious. They even come in four amazing flavors: original, moringa, cinnamon, and turmeric.

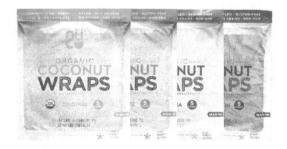

Ingredients: Organic coconut meat, organic coconut water, organic extra-virgin coconut oil. Ingredients vary depending on the flavor.

Meats and Dairy Aisle

Diestel Turkey is the number one best deli meat swap, especially when it comes to turkey. You can purchase Diestel Turkey in a package as shown below, or have it freshly cut at the deli department (what I prefer to do at our local grocer). Processed sugar, carcinogenic preservatives, and hormones typically stack up in deli meat, making it one of the most unhealthy foods out there, but with Diestel Turkey, you can rest assured you're eating clean, healthy food.

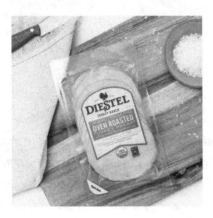

Ingredients: Organic turkey breast

Mt. Sterling Goat Cheese is melt-able, shred-able, and free of that pungent flavor found in traditional goat cheese! I cannot begin to explain how much I LOVE this cheese. You'll just have to try it on your own to find out. Even more, you can find this in a number of varieties, such as cheddar, sharp cheddar, mozzarella, pepper jack, and more!

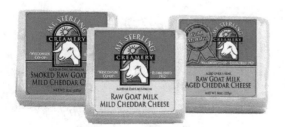

Ingredients: Cultured goat milk, salt, microbial enzymes. Ingredients vary depending on the flavor.

Natural Valley Goat Cheese is also melt-able, shred-able and mildly flavored. While I love both of these goat chesses, I've never seen them both in the same grocery store, so hopefully you will be able to find one or the other. Especially delicious, Natural Valley has mozzarella and Colby jack flavors that are perfect for kids and kids at heart.

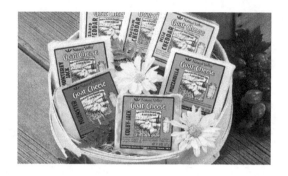

Ingredients: Pasteurized cultured goat milk, salt, enzyme. Ingredients vary depending on the flavor.

Redwood Hill Farm plain goat yogurt is my daughter's favorite yogurt swap by far. To boost sweetness and flavor, try adding a liquid stevia sweetener such as vanilla crème, blood orange, lemon, berry, or grape! Sprinkle on fresh organic berries, and you have a real treat packed with probiotics and clean protein.

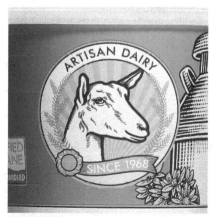

Ingredients: Pasteurized whole goat milk, tapioca, pectin, live, active cultures: S. Thermophilus, L. Bulgaricus, L. Acidophilus, Bifidus

Condiments

Organicville Ketchup has been a saving grace for my son (who is the only member of our family who really loves ketchup)! Made with agave rather than processed sugar (and most commonly, high fructose corn syrup at that), this is a must-have for any home.

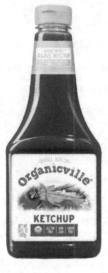

Ingredients: Organic tomato puree, organic agave nectar, organic white vinegar, salt, organic onion powder, and organic spices

Primal Kitchen Avocado Oil Mayo is a saving grace. Void of traditional inflammatory oils, it's something you can actually feel good about indulging in any recipe that calls for mayonnaise.

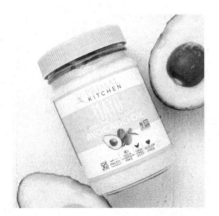

Ingredients: Avocado oil, organic cage-free eggs, organic egg yolks, organic vinegar, sea salt, rosemary extract

Organicville Tangy BBQ Sauce is a must-have for any summertime barbecue! Most barbecue sauces are full of high fructose corn syrup – which is the king of toxins when it comes to processed sugar. Similar to the brand's ketchup, Organicville Tangy BBQ sauce uses agave rather than processed sugar. Enjoy!

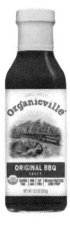

Ingredients: Organic tomato puree, organic agave nectar, organic white vinegar, organic molasses, salt, organic paprika, organic garlic powder, organic onion powder, organic minced onion, organic minced garlic, natural smoke flavor, organic chili powder, xanthan gum, organic cayenne pepper, organic cumin, organic white pepper

Primal Kitchen Ranch Salad Dressing allows you to enjoy the taste of your favorite salad dressing without eating the refined oils, dairy, sugar, and more. For years, my clients have been asking me about a good food swap for ranch dressing. Short of making my own, I have never found a good option – until now. May I present to you: Primal Kitchen's Ranch Dressing made with avocado oil!

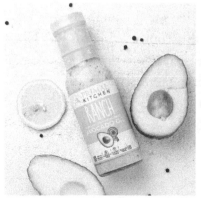

Ingredients: Avocado oil, water, organic apple cider vinegar, organic distilled vinegar, cream of tartar, sea salt, gum acacia, organic tapioca starch, organic cage-free egg powder, organic onion powder, organic garlic powder, organic lemon juice concentrate, nutritional yeast, organic parsley, konjac, organic chives, organic dill, organic black pepper, organic rosemary extract

Coconut Secret Coconut Aminos have become a secret ingredient in my kitchen. While soy sauce is another condiment that is less than ideal for our health, Coconut Secret Coconut Aminos are the perfect alternative. The taste isn't quite so strong, yet they're delicious used in a stir-fry or for a marinade on salmon or chicken breasts.

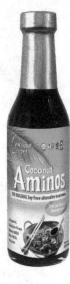

Ingredients: Organic coconut sap aged and blended with sun-dried, mineral-rich sea salt

Ice Cream Aisle

Coconut Bliss Ice Cream Sandwiches! There is nothing a kid loves more in the middle of the summer than a nice ice cream sandwich. And let's be honest, most of us adults feel the same way! However, due to the dairy, processed sugar, and, often, not-so-great preservatives, traditional ice cream sandwiches are quite inflammatory. That's why I am thrilled to share Coconut Bliss ice cream with you. Find this cookie ice cream sandwich in both a chocolate and vanilla flavor! Please do note that there's a small amount of cane sugar in the chocolate chips in these particular sandwiches.

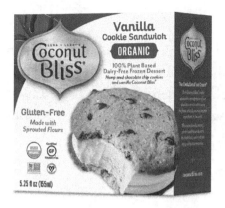

Ingredients: COCONUT MILK FROZEN DESSERT: Organic coconut milk (organic coconut, water, organic guar gum), organic agave syrup, organic coconut cream, organic vanilla extract. GLUTEN FREE COOKIES: Organic sprouted brown rice flour, organic coconut oil, organic agave syrup, organic fair trade dark chocolate chips (organic fair trade cocoa liquor, organic fair trade cane sugar, organic fair trade cocoa butter, organic fair trade cocoa powder), organic tapioca flour, organic hemp seeds, organic coconut sugar, organic millet, organic sprouted oat flour, organic applesauce, sea salt, organic flax seed, organic vanilla extract, organic guar gum, organic cinnamon, organic nutmeg

Coconut Bliss ice cream, boasting over 23 flavors, is sure to have you covered! Made with coconut milk and coconut sugar, these taste, surprisingly, *not* coconut-y! Swap out Ben and Jerry's for a scoop of your favorite flavor, and savor the idea that you can have your ice cream and eat it too, anti-inflammatory style!

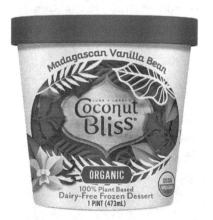

Ingredients: Organic coconut milk (organic coconut, water, organic guar gum), organic agave syrup, organic coconut cream, organic vanilla extract, organic vanilla beans. Ingredients vary depending on the flavor.

Beverage Aisle

Califia Unsweetened Almond Milk is an almond milk that comes in a convenient container, but unlike others that you may find lining the alternative milk aisle, Califia boasts fewer preservatives, as it is found in the refrigerator section rather than dry storage. As always, some options have processed sugar, so be sure to read the ingredients.

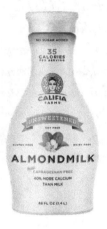

Ingredients: Almond milk (water, almonds), calcium carbonate, sunflower lecithin, sea salt, potassium citrate, natural flavors, locust bean gum, gellan gum

Califia Farms Better Half Creamer! I know parents will get as excited about an anti-inflammatory coffee creamer as kids do about ice cream. In fact, the number one comment I hear from adults, when they have swapped out cow dairy from their diet, is that they just can't quite seem to kick coffee creamer. Califia Better Half is the perfect swap that provides a natural and subtle sweetness along with the perfect rich texture. Part almond milk and part coconut milk, it's oh-so-delicious!

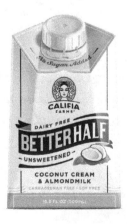

Ingredients: Almond milk (water, almonds), coconut cream, natural flavors, calcium carbonate, sunflower lecithin, monk fruit juice concentrate, sea salt, potassium citrate, locust bean gum, gellan gum

Spindrift Sparkling Water is a refreshing swap for sparking water drinks typically "enhanced" with artificial flavors. Spindrift even takes it a step further, using fruit puree for clean, crisp, all-natural flavor. It's the perfect drink for any summer barbecue or rafting trip, and comes in a number of flavors, such as raspberry lime, cucumber, grapefruit, lemon, and more.

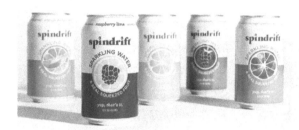

Ingredients: Sparkling water, raspberry puree, raspberry juice, fresh lime juice

GT's Kombucha is truly the only kombucha I drink. It's not only delicious but it's also free of processed sugar (post-fermentation process), whereas many kombucha companies add more processed sugar post-fermentation. Best of all, GT has fun and high vibe flavors like Lavender Love, Watermelon Wonder, Guava Goddess, and more. Come check out these healthy beverage swaps. I hope you enjoy them as much as I do!

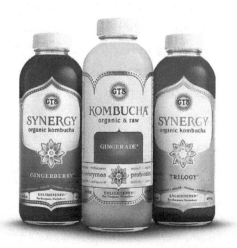

Ingredients: Raw organic kombucha, organic blueberry juice, organic ginger juice. Ingredients vary depending on the flavor.

Ancient Nutrition Bone Broth Protein simply cannot be missed in this list of grocery store swaps. Full of protein and collagen that support a healthy gut biome, the liver's detoxification process, and optimal joint function, this is a powerfully healthy drink. Add it to your smoothie, or drink it in a shaker cup. There are a number of delicious flavors to choose from!

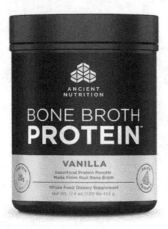

Ingredients: Non-GMO raised chicken bone broth protein concentrate, natural vanilla flavor, xantham gum, guar gum, stevia extract, and monk fruit extract

CONGRATULATIONS! You've successfully navigated the aisles of the grocery store without settling for inflammatory foods. This resource can be referred to while you are physically walking the grocery aisles, or as a support to make your next grocery list. Amazingly enough, there are still quite a few more delicious, anti-inflammatory grocery store swaps that I want to tell you about. (I've really just touched the tip of the iceberg here.) To see a comprehensive list of anti-inflammatory grocery store swaps, visit www.cleanfoodswaps.com.

With love, health, and vitality,

Jenny Carr

Further Reading

Sugar Has 56 Names: A Shopper's Guide by Robert Lustig, MD

The Real Truth About Sugar: A Full Summary and Analysis of Dr. Robert Lustig's Video Lecture "Sugar: The Bitter Truth" by Samantha Quinn

Pure, White, and Deadly: How Sugar Is Killing Us and What We Can Do to Stop It by John Yudkin

The Blood Sugar Solution: The UltraHealthy Program for Losing Weight, Preventing Disease, and Feeling Great Now! by Mark Hyman, MD

Eat Fat, Get Thin: Why the Fat We Eat Is the Key to Sustained Weight Loss and Vibrant Health by Mark Hyman, MD

The Real Food Diet Cookbook: Delicious Real Recipes for Losing Weight, Feeling Great, and Transforming Your Health by Dr. Josh Axe

Hidden Secrets to Curing Your Chronic Disease: Real Science, Real Solutions and Real Stories of Healing and Hope by Dr. Jason West

Healthy Aging: A Lifelong Guide to Your Well-Being by Andrew Weil, MD

Thank YOU!

Find out about ALL of the current and NEW anti-inflammatory grocery store swaps available to you. If you can believe it, the grocery store swaps in this book are just a fraction of the plethora of companies and foods available to you and your family! **Visit www. cleanfoodswaps.com for a complete compilation of ALL of the anti-inflammatory grocery store swaps out there!**

You will even have the opportunity to download a free guide to help you make grocery shopping super quick and easy, while choosing foods that help your family feel great (and taste delicious)!

With love,
Jenny Carr

P.S. Please accept my very special invitation to join me and my tribe on Facebook at *https://www.facebook.com/thecleaneatingkid/*

About the Author

Jenny Carr is a speaker, mom-preneur, leading inflammation expert, and the international bestselling author of *Peace of Cake: The Secret to an Anti-Inflammatory Diet*. She survived a near-death experience due to an autoimmune condition, is healing through upholding anti-inflammatory living, and is on a mission to help others do the same.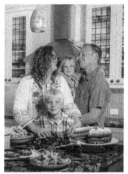

Whether it is recovering from an autoimmune disease, reversing chronic physical disorders, or easing behavioral and emotional conditions, Jenny specializes in helping people reverse these chronic symptoms by adopting and maintaining anti-inflammatory eating without feeling deprived or overwhelmed. Think cupcakes, pizza, bread, and muffins – the anti-inflammatory way!

She offers limited VIP coaching as well as her famous ***Have It ALL!*** group coaching program. Jenny has been featured by major media sources such as NBC, ABC, iHeart Radio, Dr. Mark Hyman, *US News & World Report*, Rancho La Puerta, MindBodyGreen, Well + Good, and many more.

Jenny enjoys playing, working, and living in the mountains. She resides in Jackson Hole, Wyoming, with her husband Brock and their kids Tosh and Chloe.

Endnotes

Chapter 1 - The Cost

1 "Three Hidden Ways Wheat Makes You Fat" web page, Mark Hyman, MD, February 13, 2012, https://drhyman.com/blog/2012/02/13/three-hidden-ways-wheat-makes-you-fat/

2 "Body Burden: The Pollution in Newborns" web page, EWG (Environmental Working Group), July 14, 2005, https://www.ewg.org/research/body-burden-pollution-newborns

Chapter 2 - The Magic Answer

3 "So Depression Is an Inflammatory Disease, But Where Does the Inflammation Come From?" web page, BioMed Central, U. S. National Library of Medicine, National Institutes of Health, September 12, 2013, Michael Berk, Lana J. Williams, Felice N. Jacka, Adrienne O'Neal, Julie A. Pasco, Steven Moylan, Nicholas B. Allen, Amanda L. Stuart, Amie C. Hayley, Michelle L. Byrne, and Michael Maes, https://www.ncbi.nlm.nih.gov/pmc/articles/PMC3846682/

Chapter 3 – The Secret Recipe

4 "The Vulnerable Child–Chronic Illness in US Children" web page, Focus for Health, infographic, 2015, https://www.focusforhealth.org/wp-content/uploads/2015/09/FFH-004-infographic.pdf

5 "The Sugar Timeline" web page, Hippocrates Institute, September 9, 2016, https://hippocratesinst.org/the-sugar-timeline

6 "Sugar: A Timeline" web page, an online historical timeline companion to the film, Sugar Coated: How the Food Industry Seduced the World One Spoonful at a Time, released in 2015, http://sugarcoateddoc.com/sug-

ar-timeline/

7   "Big Sugar's Sweet Little Lies: How the Industry Kept Scientists from Asking: Does Sugar Kill?" web page, Mother Jones, November/December, 2012 issue, Gary Taubes, Cristin Kearns Couzens, https://www.motherjones.com/environment/2012/10/sugar-industry-lies-campaign/

Chapter 4 – Be the Change (in Your Child's Health)

8   "Maslow's Hierarchy of Needs" web page, SimplyPsychology, Saul McLeod, updated 2018, https://www.simplypsychology.org/maslow.html

Chapter 6 – Sugar: It Makes a Difference

9   "Effect of Dietary Sugar Intake on Biomarkers of Subclinical Inflammation: A Systematic Review and Meta-Analysis of Intervention Studies" web page, PMC, U.S. National Library of Medicine, National Institutes of Health, May 12, 2018, Karen W. Della Corte, Ines Perrar, Katharina J. Penczynski, Lukas Schwingshackl, Christian Herder, Annette E. Buyken, https://www.ncbi.nlm.nih.gov/pmc/articles/PMC5986486/

10 "Sugar Addiction: Pushing the Drug-Sugar Analogy to the Limit" web page, PubMed, U.S. National Library of Medicine, National Institutes of Health, July, 2013, S. H. Ahmed, K. Guillem, Y. Vandaele, https://www.ncbi.nlm.nih.gov/pubmed/23719144

Chapter 10 – Going Deeper: Food Swaps for the Top Six Inflammatory Foods

11 "Make Sure Your Wine Is Natural – Dry Farms Wine Review" web page, This Organic Girl, April 27, 2018, Lisa Fennessy, https://thisorganicgirl.com/make-sure-your-wine-is-natural-dry-farms-wine-review/

12 "Roundup's Toxic Chemical Glyphosate, Found in 100% of California Wines Tested" web page, Healthy Holistic Living, July 9, 2016, Joseph Mercola, https://www.healthy-holistic-living.com/roundups-toxic-chemical-glyphosate-found-100-california-wines-tested/?utm_source=JERF&fbclid=IwAR1ZXpLWUzU5r1HyzwvrknmycEnJ1QtxtvRBV4vUKnbV-OwdfuHGyd8tPYw

13 "Study: 30% of Kids Have Two Or More Sugary Drinks a Day" web page, Healthy Living Matters, January 26, 2017, https://www.healthylivingmatters.net/cms/One.aspx?portalId=59296&pageId=6749925

Grocery Store Food Swaps

14 "EWG's 2019 Shopper's Guide to Pesticides in Produce" web page, EWG (Environmental Working Group), March 20, 2019, https://www.ewg.org/foodnews/summary.php

15 "Don't Want to Eat Pruitt's Pesticide? Here's What to Avoid" web page, EWG (Environmental Working Group), April 4, 2017, Alex Formuzis, Senior VP of Communications and Strategic Campaigns, Sonya Lunder, Former Senior Analyst, https://www.ewg.org/planet-trump/2017/04/don-t-want-eat-pruitt-s-pesticide-here-s-what-avoid

Printed in the USA
CPSIA information can be obtained
at www.ICGtesting.com
JSHW011057290824
69014JS00006B/135